ARTHRITIS CAN BE CURED

*A layman's guide
to the most
effective medical treatment
and cure of
arthritis, rheumatism,
neuralgia and
allied conditions.*

ARTHRITIS CAN BE CURED

BERNARD ASCHNER M.D.

FORMER CHIEF OF THE OUTPATIENT-DEPARTMENT

FOR ARTHRITIS AT STUYVESANT POLYCLINIC AND

LEBANON HOSPITALS, NEW YORK

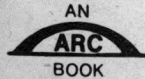
AN ARC BOOK

ARCO PUBLISHING COMPANY, INC.
219 Park Avenue South, New York, N.Y. 10003

Sixth Printing, 1977

Published by Arco Publishing Company, Inc.
219 Park Avenue South, New York, N. Y. 10003,
by arrangement with The Julian Press, Inc.

ISBN 0-668-01764-3

Printed in the United States of America

To my dear brothers
FELIX *and* CARLOS ASCHNER
in gratitude.

PREFACE

This book, which might well be entitled *Practical Relief for the Arthritic or Rheumatic Patient,* presents in simple, readily understood language the results of the author's experience over more than forty years in the treatment of literally thousands of cases of arthritis and such allied painful conditions as "rheumatism," sciatica, "lumbago," neuritis, and neuralgia. His success in obtaining comparatively prompt and long-lasting relief—often for many years—attests to the basic soundness of his concepts.

The author is an ardent student of the history of medicine; in his search into the past he has found ancient procedure so fundamentally rational and effective that it is difficult to understand why they were discarded and practically forgotten during the past hundred years. By using the best of these ancient principles and combining them with some of the physiologically sound of the more recent scientific developments, the author is convinced that arthritis is one of the most gratifying conditions to treat, because of the almost universal beneficial results obtained.

In a number of encyclopedic scientific volumes on Constitutional Therapy, the author, Dr. Bernard Aschner, has shared his knowledge and experience with the medical profession. In these pages he has made this information available in simple form to the sufferers from arthritis, not with the idea of advocating self-diagnosis and treatment, but so that the patient can, to a degree at least, understand his problem, and seek the help he needs from his doctor.

Many physicians, both in Europe and here in America, have familiarized themselves with Dr. Aschner's methods, and have treated case after case with the same almost spectacular prompt improvement, often with apparently permanent relief.

Every patient suffering from arthritis or "rheumatism" will find in these pages much valuable information to help him understand one or more of the underlying factors causing his condition. He will learn how to avoid certain mistakes in his way of life that contribute to the progress of his disease. And he will discover that, with the help of his own physician in carrying out the suggested therapeutic procedures recommended by Dr. Aschner and described in his textbook on arthritis, he can feel almost assured of a much more comfortable, useful, and happy life.

It is because of my own conviction from experience of the value of the measures advocated by the author—measures that have passed the test of time—that I have been more than happy to write these brief introductory comments, in the hope that many of the sufferers from arthritis will read these pages and benefit as a result.

NEW YORK, N.Y.   LAWRENCE W. SMITH, M.D.

CONTENTS

Physical therapy
Massage
Chiropractic and osteopathy
Radiation with X-rays
Injections
Internal medication
Orthopedic and surgical treatment

PART III

HISTORICAL SURVEY

PART ONE

GENERAL DISCUSSION

1 Widespread confusion about the cause and cure of arthritis

Incidence of arthritis and allied diseases

It is public knowledge that we have in the United States today more than ten million persons suffering from arthritis and its allied rheumatic disorders. There seems to have arisen an unfortunate pessimism about the possibility of a cure for these unhappy sufferers. The general conception is that such victims have no choice but to accept and to live with their affliction the best way they can. Modern medicine has openly stated: "We do not know what arthritis is. Therefore we have no effective cure for it."

But in this very admission lies the fundamental error of current medical thought. The whole history of medical practice reveals that medicine has often cured long before it has fully understood. Cardiac treatment, for example, discloses just such a pattern. Successful treatment of heart diseases preceded by many years total understanding of their cause. Digitalis has been used for a hundred and seventy-five years and no physician questions that it is, even today, the best heart stimulant. Doctors still have no exact idea as to how it works, however.

Modern methods have made possible many important medical advances, particularly in the treatment of infectious diseases. The fact that the chronic diseases, arthritis among them, have largely continued to defy the laboratory techniques does not necessarily make them incurable. For science to swing violently to this one-sided approach represents both a dangerous and a wasteful attitude. Medicine can not afford to disregard the many successful remedies, now relegated to the "unscientific" past, which have emerged out of practical experience, good diagnosis, observation, and even accidental cures. Scientific proof may not, as yet, have justified their usefulness. Nevertheless, they remain useful. The fundamental purpose of medicine, we must remember, is to heal, to heal as gently, as quickly, and as effectively as possible with whatever remedies we find successful.

My own more than forty years of experience, both here and in Europe, with an aggregate of about ten thousand patients suffering from arthritis, rheumatism, and allied conditions, have led me to an intensive re-examination of the past. What I have found has enabled me to cure thousands of sufferers whom the modern techniques could not, in most cases, even relieve. It has also led me to the conviction that medicine today, if it is to succeed at all with the Number One problem of chronic diseases, must achieve a synthesis in its understanding and methodology. Integration of the practical, empirical ways of the past with the modern, analytic approach may yet give us the "miracle cures" we are still searching for in chronic disease treatment.

The "miracles" I present in this book are actual case histories of patients who came to me suffering from every conceivable kind of arthritis or related disorder. I describe them with full details as to clinical symptoms, specific treatment, and exact therapeutic results. It is my hope that their documentation and my explanation of the theories on which I based my successful treatment will shed new light on the problem of arthritis, both for the unhappy victim and for the often equally unhappy practitioner who is struggling to help him.

I have said that my purpose in writing this book is to shed some light on the problem of arthritis, to prove that, contrary to current popular misconceptions, arthritis *can* be cured, and to *show how a successful cure can be achieved.* First of all, however, I feel that it is important to clear up some of the misinformation that is demoralizing and leading to the exploitation of many arthritis sufferers today.

Over a major network recently a noted radio commentator, discussing arthritis with the author of a best-selling book on the subject, disposed of the problem very simply. "People who have arthritis," he said, "just have to suffer. One can do nothing about it." This, of course, is an erroneous idea, contributing unnecessarily to the confusion of the unfortunate arthritis victim and leaving the way open to dangerous consequences for him. Panaceas, cure-alls, books, and bottles extending hope to the hopeless are quick to follow on the heels of such statements. From the doctor, the patient turns to the fringes of the medical profession, to the chiropractors, the osteopaths, the creators of diets, and writers of best-selling books about diets and other such unfounded methods of help.

Diet is one of the favorite recommendations. It is naïve, beautifully oversimplified. It promises the patient a cure "right in his own home," and without need for either doctor or medication. How eagerly our discouraged and disappointed arthritics—some even made neurotic by their many years of suffering—turn to such a hope! A forlorn hope, alas!

One of the recent best-sellers was based on the primitive and arbitrary theory that arthritis is mainly a lack of lubrication or oil in the joints. Consequently, all that the arthritic patient had to do was to provide himself with the lacking "oils" in the joints through a specific diet recommended by the author. "But what," ask I, the humble man of medicine, "what about the frequent pain and swelling in the surrounding nerves, capsules, muscles, tendons?" These the author of the book neither mentions nor explains.

He urges, instead, that his diet cure should be carried on for about half a year or perhaps a year, when results will begin to be seen. I'm afraid that very few patients would be satisfied to wait this long while under medical treatment. More often, they leave medical care if definite improvement cannot be felt within the first two to four weeks.

But to go on about this diet. . . . It permits the patient to eat fairly regular food but, strangely enough, forbids olive oil. On the other hand, a glass of milk with every one of the three meals is recommended. Now milk, we know from medical experience, disagrees with many persons, particularly the person with a weak and hyperacid stomach. Milk creates gas, more acid, constipation and, according to its chemical properties, slows down the whole process of digestion. Milk is fine for the baby; it is not always as good for the grown-up. I will discuss all this more completely in a later section on diets in arthritis. For the moment, I want to say only that I have professionally observed patients who have followed this widely publicized diet conscientiously for more than a year. They have lost strength and weight and have become anemic. In spite of the daily intake of cod-liver oil and wheat germ, also recommended in the book, their arthritis has become worse rather than better. So much for the latest popular—and perilous —fad for the cure of arthritis.

2 *An effective cure of arthritis is available*

I shall not go too much into any detailed classifications of the various forms of arthritis. For the layman, it is sufficient to know that there are only two forms of chronic arthritis as it occurs in everyday life. These are the so-called rheumatoid arthritis and the osteoarthritis.

Rheumatoid arthritis

It must be pointed out at the start that the significance of the rheumatoid, and probably infectious, type of arthritis has been unduly overemphasized in the last decade. The discovery of the "wonder drug," cortisone, and the claims made for the quick, safe, and lasting cures that could be achieved through cortisone, had a great deal to do with this. Rheumatoid arthritis, however, concerns only a very small minority, at most 5 to 10 per cent of all arthritis cases. It affects younger people, principally. As for the healing effect of cortisone, there was, at first, great enthusiasm for it; its discoverer, Dr. Hench of the Mayo Clinic, received the Nobel Prize. But the high hopes have over the years become dimmed with considerable disappointment. True, large doses of cortisone given to handicapped arthritis patients may enable them to use their arms and legs and to move around within the next few days, in an apparently amazing way. Unfortunately, the pain, stiffness, swelling, and inflammation come back after a few days, as soon as the intake of the drug is interrupted, often in an aggravated degree. The drug must be administered permanently. And its after- and side-effects are often very dangerous. High blood pressure, moonshine face (accumulation of fat and water in the soft parts of the face), abnormal hair growth on women's faces, heart disease, mental depression, and quite a number of other unpleasant and even dangerous, sometimes fatal, symptoms may develop.

There are rumors that the Mayo Clinic, the center with the largest experience in the field, may actually be abandoning the use of cortisone. I have heard one such story from a reliable physician whose patient, suffering with arthritis of the spine, returned from the Mayo Clinic stating that he had received only the orthodox therapy of heat and aspirin without, of course, any significant results.

Effective cures for rheumatic arthritis do exist, however. They are cures that give lasting results and are not dangerous. I shall discuss these, too, in a later section.

Osteoarthritis

The overwhelming majority of individuals complaining of arthritic symptoms today are not suffering from rheumatoid arthritis. They belong, rather, to the group medically classified as osteoarthritis.

This type of arthritis usually affects middle-aged or elderly persons. Here, too, many theories have been expounded, most of them leading to unjustified pessimism. The common expressions associated with osteoarthritis in recent years have been such negative ones as "degenerative," "destructive," or "progressive" arthritis, or arthritis caused simply by the "inevitable wear and tear of aging." Even if apparently supported by anatomical findings and X rays, the prognosis need not be as hopeless as these symptoms seem to indicate.

There is a cure for osteoarthritis. It is an old, old cure, discovered in antiquity. It was the classic cure up until a hundred years ago. It was, and still is, a highly satisfactory cure. It allows us the scope and practicability of direct help.

This cure is based on the knowledge that beginning with approximately the age of forty, irritant metabolic waste products such as uric acid may develop in the system and cause pain, swelling, and stiffness. If the waste products settle in the joints, the disease is called arthritis; if they accumulate in the nerves, the illness is known as neuritis or neuralgia; if they attack the soft parts of the body, the patient is suffering from rheumatism. Actually, the process is one and the same and responds very well to the same kind of treatment.

What is the best treatment for arthritis and allied conditions? The simple, logical, and practical answer is: elimination of those irritant metabolic waste products.

How can the elimination be accomplished? In two ways: first, through the outer surface, the skin; second, through the inner surface, the bowels.

3 *Cases from a physician's notebook*

Before explaining the scientific concepts underlying these theories, I would like to present some case histories. They are patients' histories, out of my own physician's notebook. They cover a private and clinical practice of more than forty years. During that time I have successfully treated thousands of cases of arthritis, rheumatism, sciatica, etc.; the documentation of these cases is available for any responsible member of the medical profession.

The cases in this volume have been selected at random to highlight specific types of conditions.

Arthritis of the wrist cured within a week

Case 1. In 1923, I went, at Christmastime, to the famous winter resort of Kitzbuehel, in the Tirol, to do some skiing. All the hotels were full. I had to be satisfied with emergency quarters in the home of an elderly country tailor. From my registration papers, he identified me as a physician. The next morning, he approached me timidly to ask for medical advice. He showed me his right wrist. It was swollen, painful, and stiff. For more than a year he had been unable to work. The diagnosis of osteoarthritis, obvious from both the symptoms and the age of the tailor, was evidently the diagnosis also reached at the Surgical University Clinic in Innsbruck, where the tailor was being treated with heat, massages, and aspirin. The treatment had not helped. I decided to try something else.

I went to the nearest drugstore and bought a piece of blistering plaster of Spanish fly (cantharides). I put this on the sore spot. After twenty-four hours a large blister, the size and shape of a watchglass, had formed. When I opened it, about a tablespoonful of yellow fluid (serum) trickled out. The patient felt immediate relief. I dressed the sore spot with a pad of gauze and a little vaseline. After five days, the skin was healed. I also prescribed small, nonlaxative amounts of calomel to be taken for one week only. Calomel is the mildest preparation of mercury, the "tamer of arthritis," some of our medical classicists call it.

By the end of one week only, the wrist, incapacitated for more than a year, was free from all distressing symptoms. The tailor was able to resume his work. He never forgot his gratitude. Each year, up until 1938 when I left Vienna, he sent me his Christmas card, telling me about his appreciation and, what was more important medically, his continued well-being.

Sciatica cured within a week

Case 2. In 1908, when I was getting my postgraduate training in Vienna at the famous Surgical University Clinic of Professor von Eiselsberg, I also had a number of private patients. One of these was a very wealthy woman who had been suffering for more than a year from an extremely stubborn and painful sciatica. She had visited the most exclusive health resorts in Europe, consulted the best specialists in Vienna, all without relief. I, too, had at that time no help to give her.

But I knew that Dr. Frantisek Jetel, a Czech physician, was then practicing in Vienna. He attracted large crowds of patients suffering from arthritis, rheumatism, and allied conditions whom he cured rapidly with a rash-producng ointment, the composition of which he kept a secret. His "secret" had earned him the dislike of the medical profession. I saw no harm in suggesting to my patient, after telling her the facts, that she might consult Dr. Jetel. I went with her.

Dr. Jetel, a sturdy, self-reliant man, looked briefly at the patient, and without using any instrument or test, laconically said in his Czech dialect, "Madam will be cured in a week." I was more than surprised; I was highly skeptical. But Dr. Jetel proceeded with his treatment. He rubbed a sharply aromatic-smelling ointment over the whole painful area. He repeated this on three successive days. He also ordered the patient to wear for one week a special kind of course, cotton underwear, which he kept ready for such use.

By the end of the third day, a dense, scarletlike, painless rash, consisting of small pimples each the size of a millet grain, had appeared. The rash dried up within a week. The sciatica pain was gone for good. I observed this patient professionally for many years afterward. She never suffered a relapse.

Quick cure of neuralgia of the arm

Case 3. Then there was the case of my lawyer whom I met one day in 1932, on a street in Vienna. He was wearing his arm in a black sling. I asked him whether he had been in an accident. In a desperate voice, he told me that he had been suffering for more than six weeks from a most painful neuralgia of his right arm. He had just come from Court. Unable to write his signature, he had had to make three crosses, like an illiterate. He suffered sleepless nights, despite large doses of morphine. His family physician had called in a nerve specialist. Certain protein injections, medically fashionable at the time, had been prescribed. The nerve specialist had told him, however, that no one could really say how long the disease would last. It might be months before he could use his arm again.

I got in touch with his family physician. We applied an artificial rash with the use of a liniment recommended in the old textbooks —perhaps this was Dr. Jetel's cure—over the whole painful area. Within a week, the rash dried up and the neuralgia was gone. It never came back.

Arthritis of the knees quickly cured

Case 4. More recently, I treated a number of Catholic priests and nuns who could no longer kneel down in church because of chronic arthritis (osteoarthritis) of the knees. The condition had been going on in some cases for months, in others for years. Present-day treatment had not been able to help them. My associates and I applied several plasters of Spanish fly once or twice a week in succession, until pain, swelling, and stiffness were completely gone. The treatment was combined with medication for the cause of the stiffness, the deposits in the arthritic joints. Overweight pointed to an overcharged metabolism. A reducing cure, consisting of a low caloric diet, thyroid tablets, and saline laxatives was prescribed. Within a few weeks, these patients appeared permanently freed from their distress.

4 The external and internal treatment of arthritis

◆

Draining of the skin by counter-irritation or blistering

And what conclusions may we draw from these and countless other case histories that follow the same pattern? We may safely say that draining of the skin by producing counter-irritation or blistering is a method that gives the quickest and most gratifying results in the treatment of osteoarthritis. It serves to eliminate the irritant metabolic waste products through the outer surface of the skin. The treatment is fully discussed in earlier medical texts. It is described under the scientific name of the exanthematic method, exanthema meaning rash or skin eruption. It can be applied in all the allied illnesses—sciatica of the legs, neuralgia of the arms, the head, the face, and of the intercostal areas, corresponding to the nerves that run along the ribs.

The cure of arthritis by internal medication

Since the earliest days arthritis, at that time called "podagra" or "chronic gout," has been treated successfully by the various methods of blistering and by specific antiarthritic internal medication. These specific medicines for arthritis consisted then of various herbs (e.g., burdock root and colchicum, which is meadow saffron), also certain resins (such as aloes), and later on chemicals, even metals such as gold, mercury, and antimony. One of these specific antiarthritic compositions was particularly effective and bore the significant name, "Holy Bittrs." It contained the resins of aloes, scammonium, and agaricus. Similar compounds were used up until a hundred years ago under such characteristic names as "antirheumatic liquor," "antipodagric pills," or "antipodagric powder." The latter is a mild and harmless, though effective, compound of gold to be taken by mouth.

I have collected much of this knowledge and described it in my scientific textbook, *Treatment of Arthritis and Rheumatism in General Practice,* the Froben Press, New York, 1946.

I should like now to describe a striking example of such a cure through a "secret" internal medicine.

Multiple arthritis (polyarthritis) cured by a herb potion

Case 5. In 1922, I was asked to treat the wife of the Austrian Minister of Commerce for a condition of too scanty menstruation. But, at the same time, she complained of a steadily progressive arthritis in various joints. Her fingers, knees, shoulders, and elbows had become painful, swollen, stiff, and cracking. She had consulted the best specialists of Vienna. Some of them wanted her to have her tonsils taken out; others advised extraction of her beautiful teeth.

At that time there were rumors of a famous lay healer, a peasant who lived in the provincial town of Graz, in Styria. He had cured many hundreds of patients by a secret potion, which he prepared himself and gave directly to the sick, then coming to him from all parts of Europe. My patient asked my consent to consult this lay healer. She went there for three weeks, came back to me free from all complaints. She was able to attend her dancing parties, her Sunday trips, and all the other social obligations of a minister's wife, as if she had never had arthritis at all.

She brought back with her a bottle of her medicine, a kind of white wine that had a bitter aftertaste, apparently the effect of the bitter herb used as an ingredient. Every expert knows how difficult and often even impossible it is to identify such herbs by chemical analysis unless they contain certain characteristic elements such as the well-known alkaloids or glycosides, digitalis, strychnine, morphine, belladonna, and the like. I could only guess at the contents. But I found, again in the old textbooks, a bitter-tasting herb that would meet the requirements of a remedy for arthritis. It was herba gratiolae (Herb of Mercy), used by one of the greatest medical practitioners who ever lived, namely Hufeland, Goethe's personal physician and also professor in Jena and Berlin until the early part of the nineteenth century.

Several other such antiarthritic and antirheumatic drugs in the form of herbs and their extracts or in the form of chemicals are also described in my scientific textbook and can still be applied usefully by any modern physician.

The two-way treatment of arthritis

Paracelsus, the famous physician of the sixteenth century, considered almost a magician because of his seemingly unbelievable curative powers, who stated that pain can be removed from a painful spot by blistering of the skin, also said: "Arthritis must be treated in two ways, from outside by draining of the skin, and from inside through the bowels." Both ways of treatment can be accomplished by a variety of internal and external drugs that were developed into a refined art by earlier masters of medicine.

Physicians treating osteoarthritis with the exanthematic methods today usually prescribe, simultaneously, the required dosage of medication for antiarthritic laxative purposes. A number of specific antiarthritic laxatives and similar drugs exist to cleanse the system of metabolic waste. Osteoarthritis is mainly a metabolic disease, like obesity, diabetes, or acute and chronic gout. This last is almost identical with osteoarthritis.

For a thorough and lasting cure

In my textbook for physicians, I have described a vast number of cures based on my methods. On the surface, they seem very simple methods and lay readers may find the idea of self-treatment a very tempting one. This is *not* recommended. *No treatment of arthritis should be attempted without a physician.*

Even the physician must be cautious. If he wants to establish a thorough and lasting cure, he must always look for the deeper causes of the metabolic disturbance, which may vary from individual to individual within certain well-defined limits. In other words, local treatment must be accompanied by correct general care.

Overweight people must reduce. People who are very thin are often suffering from chronic indigestion of the stomach. This must be promptly diagnosed and treated. The same holds true for insufficient menstruation or diminished skin perspiration. An overcharged metabolism must, in every way indicated by the individual need, be properly corrected.

Hidden treasures of medicine

At this point, the intelligent reader may indeed have a pertinent question to ask. Why are these methods of treating arthritis not in general use today? The most outstanding physicians of the past effected thousands of successful cures by using them. The author of this book and the numerous physicians in Europe who accepted and followed his theories cured a large number of cases, in both private and clinical practice. Cured patients have been presented for observation and study at medical meetings and conferences. This author's results have been published in scientific articles and textbooks. Why ignore such factual evidence, such proved experience?

The answer lies in the nature of our modern society. Fashions in medicine, unfortunately, change almost as frequently as styles in women's clothes. If a certain treatment does not seem to fit into the currently fashionable system of medicine, it is often disregarded, frequently almost fanatically written off the books as unscientific and unacceptable. In many cases, this is an unhappy error.

A new discovery, such as Dr. Salk's vaccine for infantile paralysis, for example, may be very readily accepted; it fits exactly into the line of current laboratory medicine, especially into the modern doctrine of immunization.

The successful treatment of arthritis, however, as advocated by this author, is an outgrowth of what we call our empirical medical system, a system based on the collected experience of two thousand years of medical research and practice. Knowledge rooted in such deep, continuing experience, supplemented by today's analytical laboratory techniques, may be the only way to find the "miracle" arthritis cure that so many are seeking.

5 *The great medical revolution*

Most persons outside the medical profession do not know that a revolution in medical science took place about a hundred years ago. At that time the German anatomist, Rudolf Virchow, introduced the system of "cellular pathology." In simpler, nonmedical language, this means a system of medicine based on a study of the cells or solid parts of the body that we can see under a microscope. It was Virchow's contention that cellular pathology was the only scientific method because we can control the morbid changes of the cells in the microscopic picture.

The previous system of medicine, called "humoral pathology," was based not on the pathology of the solid cells, but on the fluids or humors of the body, that is the blood, the bile, the lymph or serum, and the phlegm or mucus.

But "a man's life is in his blood," as the Bible says, or as our Latinists wrote, "corpora no agunt nisi fluida"—"matter reacts only in a fluid state." In the eighteenth century, Hunter, one of England's greatest physicians, expressed the same idea in a more scientific way, saying, "The blood is the carrier of life." Still more recently, biochemical research in the lymphatic, enzymatic, and endocrine fields goes far to prove that there is a solid foundation for major parts of the humoral theory.

Modern medicine can be proud of its recent accomplishments. But it cannot afford to be rash. It cannot throw out a collected knowledge and experience of thousands of years without actually impoverishing its own healing capacity.

Strides in modern medicine

Everyone knows that modern medicine has made enormous progress in the field of acute infectious diseases by the discovery of the sulfa drugs and of the antibiotics, such as penicillin, aureomycin, chloromycetin, and the like. These new discoveries have enabled the modern physician to succeed phenomenally in the battle against the great epidemic infectious diseases. And the nonepidemic infectious diseases, such as for example pneumonia, can also be cured more quickly and with much less danger and complication than thirty years ago.

Poor results of modern medicine in chronic diseases

On the other hand, the medical profession admits that our healing results in chronic diseases lag far behind our other accomplishments. Our daily obituary pages are full of accounts of those between the early ages of forty-five and sixty-five who die of heart attacks or of cerebral hemorrhages or strokes. Our modern physicians still treat high blood pressure, ulcer, asthma, many skin conditions, conditions of the eyes, ears, female organs, even mental diseases with methods that are long, tedious, expensive and, most important, too often, ineffective. The classic ways of treating these illnesses may not have had sufficient "scientific evidence" or "rationalistic explanations" to support them. But they generally cured more quickly and more often. As I have pointed out in my *Textbook on Constitutional-Therapy,* a radical change in our methodological approach is necessary in respect to most of our chronic diseases. A re-examination of ourselves and of the resources of our own neglected past is definitely indicated.

6 The most successful cures of arthritis by combination of the earlier with the modern medical system

This author has made it the task of his life to study the practical facts of medical history and of the medical systems of all times and nations, and to combine them with modern science and technique. It has proved to be most effective in both clinical and private practice, particularly in the cure of arthritis and its related conditions. Numerous other physicians, particularly in Europe, have confirmed the same good results over a period of more than forty years. It is to be hoped that the United States, our "young" country, ever striving toward the new, will also soon take stock of both its own headlong progress and of the sometimes more thoughtful healing arts of our medical predecessors.

Earlier textbooks reveal that many of our medical predecessors were much more successful in the treatment of arthritis than we are today. It was Paracelsus, one of the most outstanding physicians of all times, who said, "Wherever nature produces pain, there she accumulates harmful substances and wants to eliminate them. If she cannot accomplish that herself [e.g., by abscesses, hemorrhages, or skin eruptions], the physician must create an artificial outlet in order to provide an escape for these harmful products." This is one of the classic statements that make up the foundation upon which much of our medical knowledge is based. It is also the theory underlying the treatment of arthritis by draining of the skin.

I have already referred to two of the most practical ways of skin-draining or counter-irritation, as it is called today. The first is vesication, which means forming a blister by application of plaster of Spanish fly, scientifically called plaster of cantharides. The name, Spanish fly, comes to us from the Moors or Arabs who occupied Spain in the Middle Ages. They had brought the drug, cantharides powder, from the orient to Spain and introduced its use to the Europeans. Cantharides are the powdered product of a dried small greenish beetle, related to our cockchafer. It contains an irritant blistering substance, called cantharidin. This powder is mixed with resins and fat and turned into a salve or plaster. When applied for twenty-four hours on the most painful or swollen spot, it forms a blister like a watchglass. Often the pain disappears "like magic" overnight. Most often, the cure is a permanent one. The plaster of Spanish fly, usually applied in the size of one to four postage stamps, can be used on all different joints, but always combined with proper internal general care.

The second practical method of skin-draining is through the production of an artificial rash over the whole painful area. This is accomplished by rubbing into the skin, with the necessary medical precautions, of course, an irritant liniment. The main ingredient of this liniment is Croton oil, product of a tropical plant.

Most of the secret ointments used by lay healers of the past contained Croton oil mixed with various other ingredients. We may admit the same possibility about some of our more recent healers.

In Vienna, in the 1920's, a retired letter carrier sold large amounts of such a secret rash-producing liniment, probably inherited from some old relatives. The cure was so effective and he became so rich that he ended up as the landlord of four large houses.

This story belongs in the same category as the one told by members of the New York Philharmonic Symphony Society about the recently deceased conductor, Toscanini. He had been handicapped for some time by a severe arthritis of his right shoulder. He could not find any help among the modern medical practitioners in New York. He went to Dr. Munari, in Treviso, near Venice. Dr. Munari had also cured thousands of arthritic and rheumatic patients by producing an artificial rash with a secret ointment. He tried the same treatment with the conductor. After a very short time, Toscanini came back to New York free from arthritic pain. He remained free of it for the rest of his life.

Nature cures

Even the "fathers of medicine," the great Hippocrates in ancient Greece, Galen, the physician of the Roman emperors in the second century A.D., and even more so, Paracelsus in the sixteenth century admitted that they learned many practical cures from simple folk—from the peasants, the shepherds, the old herb-gathering women, the barber-surgeons, jailers, even the gypsies.

It may be that a beekeeper had, at one time, arthritis of his hands. But he was cured by bee stings, a kind of counter-irritation of the skin. This fact was confirmed later on by physicians who experimented with live bees. Bee venom, administered by injection, does not have the same effect, however.

At another time, a barefoot peasant with gout or arthritis in his feet may have stepped accidentally into an ant hill. He was bitten by the ants. The arthritis disappeared.

Or a middle-aged woman, suffering from arthritis of her hands, knees, or ankles, looking for berries or herbs in the woods, may have been touched by nettles or poison ivy. A superficial rash developed and the pain, at least to a certain extent, diminished or disappeared.

Many great discoveries in nature were made by such accidental observations. No less a man than Isaac Newton discovered the law of gravity by watching an apple falling from a tree and drawing the proper conclusions.

Baunscheidt's exanthematic blistering method

A German mechanic named Carl Baunscheidt discovered in a similar way his own successful system of blistering about a hundred years ago. He wrote a book on his experiences with the thousands of patients he had cured. His book went through numerous editions and was finally edited and revised by the German physician, Dr. Schauenstein, in the second half of the last century. Baunscheidt made his discovery in the following way:

Case 6. He had been suffering for a long time from arthritis of the right wrist. The joint was painful, swollen, and half-stiffened. He could not get any help from the "modern" medical knowledge of the time. One summer evening, he was sitting at the window of his house in Endenich, a little place on the banks of the Rhine, sadly nursing his sick hand. Swarms of mosquitoes came in from the swampy banks of the river. He let them settle down on his wrist, perhaps with the half-conscious thought of the healing effect of insect bites that I have mentioned earlier. In fact, the very next day his wrist, intensively stung by the mosquitoes, was no longer either swollen or painful. He was able to go back to work, just as the country tailor had done after the healing effect of blistering with Spanish fly.

Baunscheidt, a mechanic by profession, decided to construct a little apparatus that would imitate the insect bites. It consisted of a round metal disk, the size of a quarter, in which twenty fine sewing needles were soldered at their blunt ends. The points of the needles could be thrust into the surface of the skin by an elastic spring contraption. In this way, the superficial pores of the skin were opened without producing any bleeding. We do just about this in the case of smallpox vaccination, today. Afterwards, Baunscheidt rubbed into the pricked skin an irritant rash-producing liniment. The exact composition of this liniment was never revealed but we do know that its main ingredient was Croton oil.

Baunscheidt founded a whole school of lay healers in Germany, called the Baunscheidtists. They attracted large crowds of rheumatic and arthritic patients, who had been disappointed with regular medical care. His methods cured most of them, even such severe cases as arthritis of the spine. His treatment is still widely used in Germany, particularly by homeopathic and naturopathic physicians and also by lay healers, doubtless with much success.

The Kneipp cure

One of the most popular lay healers in Germany during the second half of the nineteenth century was the Catholic priest, Monsignor Kneipp. At a time when scientific medicine was lost in deep pessimism, almost in nihilism, and was therefore unable to help the major part of the sick, Monsignor Kneipp in a small town of Bavaria went on quietly healing with his nature cures consisting of diet, herbs, and hydrotherapy (application of cold water). He, too, applied a rash-producing secret liniment containing Croton oil and with it achieved many successful cures of arthritis, rheumatism, neuralgia, lumbago, and the like.

Even now, a whole school of scientifically trained physicians follows his principles, and the small town of Woerishofen in Bavaria belongs among the most popular health resorts of Europe today.

7   *What causes arthritis?*

❖

Local and general causative factors

I have demonstrated in previous chapters that an effective cure for arthritis definitely exists. This applies to the large majority of all arthritic cases, particularly the most frequent form, osteoarthritis, provided, naturally, that the disease is not too far advanced or neglected. I have also stated that osteoarthritis, usually, is not a mere local condition but a general disease, caused by certain metabolic disturbances. In medicine, the essential purpose of which is to cure the sick, a goal more urgent than chemical formulas or absolute laboratory research, the theories I describe are important because they lead to a safe and practical cure in a relatively short time.

A large number of both local and general factors may cause arthritis. Becoming acquainted with them may help the reader to recognize certain characteristic abnormalities of the body and also to avoid certain faulty living habits that frequently contribute to the development of arthritis.

The local causes, such as injuries or permanent strain of a joint, are less important. Examples are the tennis elbow, the golfer's arm, "housemaid's knee," a fractured hip joint, or the fallen arches of waiters, the last caused by long periods of standing on the feet, often complicated by arthritis of the surrounding joints.

The general causes of arthritis are much more numerous. I shall first enumerate them and give the explanation afterward, step by step. These general causes are: age, sex, overweight, fullness of blood, high blood pressure, overcharged metabolism (mainly uric acid diathesis), chronic indigestion of the stomach, constipation, diseases of the liver and the gall bladder, insufficient perspiration of the skin, inadequate (too rare or too scanty) menstruation, natural (and even more so artificial) menopause, and bad living habits, such as excessive smoking or drinking or a hectic, high-pressured day-to-day life.

Age and arthritis

The large majority of all cases of arthritis consists of middle-aged or elderly people. If we go to health resorts specializing in arthritis cures, we will see that they are almost exclusively patronized by these age groups. A glance into an outpatient department for arthritis will reveal the same picture.

Arthritis in the young

There are however, rather as an exception, younger people affected by arthritis, particularly young women who suffer from arthritis of the fingers. But these cases are rare, accounting for only about 5 to 10 per cent of all arthritic patients. This arthritis in younger individuals usually belongs to rheumatoid arthritis, the real cause of which is not yet fully understood. It is also called "probably infectious arthritis" because of the possibility that it may be due to infectious foci in the tonsils, teeth, or other organs. Sometimes the removal of these foci improves or cures the condition, but very often it does not. There was a period when this trend of "sanitation" was overdone, and carried out even in the noninfectious osteoarthritis. Not knowing the real causative factors at the time, the medical profession often recommended "removal" on almost a wholesale basis.

Many persons have thus unnecessarily lost their tonsils, which are important as a "watchdog" for the brain, helping to prevent infantile paralysis, for example, and as a "watchdog" for the lungs, protecting them against tuberculosis. I would not hesitate to say that the increase in the frequency of infantile paralysis in this country has been a great deal provoked by the mass hysteria of having the tonsils removed in every child, nearly as a matter of compulsory routine. The present radical enucleation of the tonsils will one day be recognized as harmful malpractice.

Even if a child has had repeated attacks of tonsilitis, removal of the tonsils is hardly ever necessary except in rare cases. This operation kills the "watchdog" instead of curing it. Repeated attacks of tonsilitis in children usually have their cause in stomach trouble, particularly in cases of incorrect nutrition and especially in cases where overfeeding of milk is a factor. Inflammation of the tonsils in children or adults can be successfully treated in a conservative way, through proper disinfectant gargles or through the more recently discovered chemotherapies and antibiotics.

Also, the fear of "silent" infection of the roots of the teeth (so-called granuloma, seen in the X-ray picture) is grossly exaggerated. A good dentist can frequently preserve the teeth with conservative treatment and the patient should fight to keep every one of them. There was a time, particularly in England, but also in this country, when one often saw young people with total artificial dentures; mass extraction of all their teeth had taken place as an alleged cure for arthritis.

Rheumatoid arthritis is today supposed to be cured in a specific way by ACTH, cortisone, and its derivatives (hydrocortisone, meticortone, etc.). But, as I have already said, the original enthusiasm has been replaced by disappointment, for the drug must be continued endlessly and, in the long run, may have many dangerous side-effects.

Actually, *rheumatoid arthritis can be cured* in a much safer way by using methods similar to the ones I have suggested for osteoarthritis, but with special emphasis on mild preparations of mercury (small doses of calomel) and of antimony. But this is a matter for physicians who may read about it in this author's scientific textbook. I mention these facts here only in order to reassure discouraged patients, so that they may know there is such a safe cure available.

Arthritis in the middle-aged and elderly

How often patients ask their physicians, "But why do I have arthritis?"! It is often difficult to make them understand that the mere process of growing older (after the age of forty), in itself results in a slowing down of the chemical processes of the body. A comparison with the motor of an old automobile that does not quite so promptly or so completely utilize its gasoline is obvious. The older the person—or the car—gets, the more refuse is produced.

Physicians know very well that very often in the later decades of life more and more metabolic waste products accumulate in the system. These waste products can best be classified under the approximate common denominator of uric acid, an approximation that provides, at the same time, the most practical way for a successful cure.

The waste products resulting from an incomplete assimilation of food may act as an irritant agent and cause all kinds of disturbances. They may cause pain in the joints, the nerves, the muscles, the tendon sheaths, and other tissues. Swelling, exudation, inflammation, and stiffness in all these parts may result. They may also provoke cramps in the coronary arteries of the heart as well as in the arteries of the whole body, thus producing high blood pressure.

All this applies to the cause of arthritis and may be aggravated by faulty living habits, as I have mentioned before.

We often read in the newspapers about persons in public life who are suffering from arthritis. Recently we have read this about a number of famous musical conductors and also about President Eisenhower, who has been suffering for several years from arthritis of the shoulder. More interesting medically, however, is the fact that most of these sufferers are middle-aged and elderly men.

8   *Sex and arthritis*

Sex is an important factor in arthritis. According to official statistics, women during the last fifty years have been affected by arthritis four to six times more often than men. In other words, more than two thirds of all arthritic patients are women, and among them, one third of all women after the menopause suffer from arthritis, to a lesser or greater degree. This startling fact can be explained by the fundamental difference between the endocrine glands of the sexes and also by the different metabolism of women. The relationship, therefore, between arthritis and the physiological functions characteristic of women, such as the rhythmic menstrual period, pregnancy, lactation, and menopause are much more complicated. I shall first discuss briefly the relationship between the male sex and arthritis.

Male sex and arthritis

Since antiquity, gout or arthritis in young men has been correctly related to a considerable degree to heredity and to sexual excesses and other debauchery. Arthritis in men after the age of forty may also be aggravated by overindulgence in sexual activities. This is frequently neither realized nor accepted by the patient. Many men suffer from wounded pride if they cannot continue to live the sexual life of a young man up to the age of sixty or even seventy and over. I have often found this so when trying to advise a male arthritic patient to be sexually abstinent at least until the arthritis was cured.

The following case history is a striking example of such a pattern:

Case 7. Some years ago, a sixty-year-old robust man, a bachelor in New York who was well to do and retired from business, came to consult me about his arthritis. He complained of violent pain and stiffness in all joints. He seemed to be in permanent agony, finding it extremely difficult to sit down, get up, or even to achieve a comfortable sleeping position.

He had already consulted a number of outstanding specialists. They had prescribed the usual remedies for gout but without any satisfactory result.

When I asked him about his living habits, he boasted that he had always had a very full life in every respect and that he was still able, in sexual matters, to conduct himself as a young man. Since he was overweight, I prescribed a reducing diet, consisting of a low caloric intake, thyroid tablets, and saline laxatives, the last to remove accumulated waste products. I also applied a mild counter-irritation or skin-blistering on the most painful areas. From the very beginning, I advised complete sexual abstinence until a cure was completed, and moderation for the future.

His condition improved rapidly. At the end of six weeks, he was completely free of complaints.

Half a year later, however, he made a kind of honeymoon

trip to Florida with a woman much younger than himself. After a few weeks, he returned to my office in the same miserable agony as he was before my treatment began.

I can report quite a number of similar cases in which it was very difficult to convince men in their seventh or eighth decade of life that they had to use moderation in their sexual activities if they wanted to be cured of arthritis. The same is true for elderly patients suffering from diseases of the heart, the stomach, or other organs. I remember a seventy-five-year-old former army officer whose hearing was deteriorating from year to year owing to a process in the ear similar to hardening of the arteries or arthritis. He insisted on conducting his married life with all the excesses of a young man, although I explained to him the risk of becoming completely deaf.

The ancients had a proverb: *Venus, potus, otium faciunt podagrum.* Love-making, wine-drinking, and laziness create podagra (arthritis). A similar old proverb reads: "Bacchus (wine) is the father, Venus the mother of gout (arthritis)." All this concerns men, but not women.

Female sex and arthritis

I have mentioned that women have a much greater disposition to arthritis than men because of the much more complicated functions of their sexual organs. Even in younger years, women suffering from arthritis almost always evidence a too rare or too scanty menstruation. This fact is often overlooked in diagnosis. Modern medicine has, in general, not been paying much attention to the fundamental significance of a regular and sufficiently strong menstruation for a woman's health. The great masters of medicine called menstruation "the sign and bulwark of health"—*signum et praesidium sanitatis.* They also considered it a most impressive and fundamentally important form of elimination, expressed by the Latin words *solemnis illa excretio.*

Any disturbance in the rhythm or quantity of this monthly "cleaning of the system" may result in a kind of autointoxication (self-poisoning) through the retention of harmful waste products meant to be eliminated.

The monthly cleaning process protects the female sex from many diseases to which men are subjected. For example, angina pectoris is much rarer in women than in men; it usually occurs only after premature artificial menopause by surgery or radiotherapy.

It is therefore a mistake to advise young females not to "coddle" themselves, to tell them they may continue their usual dancing, training, swimming, or other strenuous activities during the menstrual period. This often results in too rare or too scanty menstruation with consequent inflammations in various organs, e.g., in the eyes or in the skin, and in arthritic conditions.

Case 8. I met a very dramatic example of such misjudgment in my practice. In 1932, a very well-known young lady dancer came to consult me in my office in Vienna. She was twenty-seven years old and utterly depressed because of rapidly spreading arthritis in her fingers, knees, shoulders, and spine. This condition had begun one and a half years earlier. She had tried all the usual treatments—diathermy, short wave, injections, internal remedies, radiation with X rays, but all to no avail.

The fact that her menstruation had become too rare and too scanty because of uninterrupted training, even during the menstrual period, had been overlooked.

My patient was afraid that she would have to give up her profession and become an invalid. The best specialists had brought no relief, had even told her that the condition, particularly in the spinal area, was irresistibly progressive. She was advised to wear a heavy, harnesslike corset of steel and leather, reaching from the armpits down to the middle of the thighs, which, of course, horrified the attractive and ambitious young dancer who used to give performances all over Europe.

I proceeded, first, to correct her insufficient menstruation, which was then lasting only one and a half days instead of the previous four to five, by proper medication. I also prescribed internal specific drugs for arthritis, including small amounts of calomel, and intensive use of a sweating cabinet. My patient was restored to full health within two months. She was able to resume her profession as a dancer. With the necessary precautions, she remained well as long as I could observe her in Vienna, from 1932 to 1938.

"Blood is quite a peculiar sap," says the devilish Mephisto in Goethe's *Faust*. This applies especially to the menstrual blood, which is supposed to contain as well as to eliminate "poisonous" harmful substances. In the Middle Ages, menstrual blood was therefore used for witchcraft. In modern times the great scientist, Professor Bela Schick, originator of the famous Schick test for diphtheria and formerly Director of the Children's Clinic at Mount Sinai Hospital in New York, describes in a medical journal his experiments proving that some women, during their menstruation, exude certain toxic substances even through the skin, which make flowers touched by them fade quickly.

More important, however, are the toxinlike effects of menstrual blood if, because of insufficient elimination, it remains in the woman's body. There it may cause pain, inflammation, and swelling in any organ, and thus is a frequent contributing cause to arthritis. Two things must be done in such cases: first, one must try to bring the menstruation back to its normal strength and regularity; second, one must try to eliminate the accumulated menstrual toxins, which, of course, is a doctor's job.

Arthritis of the menopause

One may correctly use the term "arthritis of the menopause" since the three causative factors of age, sex, and lack of menstruation are all combined at this stage of life. I have already explained that middle-aged and elderly people, because of their sluggish metabolism, have a greater disposition to arthritis, that women are affected by arthritis four to six times more often than men, and that the menstrual flow is a rhythmic cleansing process important for a woman's health, not only because it is the shedding of an unimportant by-product of the monthly ovulation and of the uterine membranes connected with this process.

Such a natural change as the step from regular menstruation to menopause should occur without any disturbances in a woman's health. It was and still is the case with women living under more natural circumstances. Women in many primitive tribes, for example, peasant women, and women with particularly strong constitutions and good living habits do not usually suffer during the menopause. Under more civilized living conditions, however, the transition into the menopause does not always occur as smoothly. There are the well-known hot spells or flushes and attacks of sweating. It is commonly believed that this change of life does not usually last longer than one or two years. But very often such flushes and sweats last for many years, sometimes even for the remainder of the lifetime. They are just the most superficial symptoms, indicating that the whole metabolism and circulation are deeply changed. Every stage of life has different physiological laws and characteristic chemical processes with special tendencies to different diseases.

In reference to the menopause, classic medicine states that female bodies are affected by three dispositions: (1) obesity or overweight, (2) fullness of blood, of which the heat spells are a symptom, and (3) a typical metabolic disturbance characterized by an overcharging of the body with irritant metabolic waste products closely related to uric acid. This explains the high frequency of arthritis in women after the menopause.

Good treatment of the menopause, therefore, cannot consist only of the prescribing of hormones and sedatives; it must correct the three factors mentioned above, namely overweight, fullness of blood, and overcharged metabolism.

Premature artificial menopause and arthritis

Observation of a large number of women patients has taught most doctors that even *spontaneous premature menopause,* between the ages of thirty-six and forty-six, as sometimes happens in women with weak endocrine glands, may provoke symptoms of a stormy change of life, among them mental depression, palpitations of the heart, high blood pressure—and arthritis.

The results are often even more serious if the menstruation is suddenly interrupted by surgery, radium, or X rays long before the age of the natural menopause, which is in the temperate zone at about fifty years. Premature artificial menopause is usually brought on by severe hemorrhage or by tumors of the uterus (mostly fibroids, also called myomas) or of the ovaries in the form of cysts. A radical procedure is, of course, necessary in the case of cancer which, fortunately is not as frequent by far as recent publicity has led us to believe.

A physician realizing the importance of regular menstruation for a woman's health will make every effort to preserve it up to the age of the natural menopause. In cases of severe hemorrhage without a tumor, it is almost always possible to correct the condition by proper general care and by certain well-established remedies for stopping the hemorrhage. Sometimes minor surgery (such as curettage of the uterine membrane) or the insertion of a styptic pencil of zinc chloride into the uterine cavity will accomplish the purpose.

The most frequent cause for surgical removal of the uterus (hysterectomy) is fibroids. The gynecologist who believes in the importance of preserving the menstruation can, in the large majority of cases, peel these tumors out of their bed in the uterine wall. By a kind of plastic operation, he may then retain enough substance in the sound part of the uterus to make possible a sufficient and regular menstrual flow. A number of American and European gynecologists, this author among them, have advocated and practiced this type of conservative myomectomy with good success. In America, the radical hysterectomy is usually preferred, largely because of the exaggerated fear of cancer in the remaining part of the uterus. One of the very few American gynecologists who perform the conservative myomectomy is Dr. I. C. Rubin, discoverer of the famous Rubin Test for sterility and formerly Chief of the Gynecological Department at New York's Mount Sinai Hospital. Dr. Rubin definitely believes that women after a conservative myomectomy feel much better than those who have undergone radical hysterectomy.

Not all women suffer severely after premature artificial menopause. Among the most frequent symptoms, when they suffer, are high blood pressure, heart disease, mental depression, overweight, and particularly a tendency to severe forms of arthritis, including generalized arthritis (polyarthritis), involving numerous joints, and also a specific arthritis of the spine. Even the last condition, as I shall describe in a later chapter, can be successfully treated by the methods advocated in this book.

9 Obesity as a frequent causative factor in arthritis

Whenever an overweight patient suffering from arthritis enters my office, I am rather confident that I can promise a rather rapid and substantial recovery if the patient co-operates in carrying out my reducing cure. Certain diseases such as anemia, avitaminosis, etc. are caused by a deficiency of important bodily substances; others such as arthritis, may come as a result of a surplus of material owing to fullness of blood, overweight, or overcharged metabolism.

As soon as we rid ourselves of the currently pessimistic notion that the cause of arthritis must still be sought somewhere in the clouds or in some yet unborn, mysterious laboratory research and as soon as we accept the cause of arthritis as the surplus of waste products, we easily understand that overweight and an thritis, both surplus diseases, are as closely related as members of a family. Incidentally, one glance into an arthritis clinic confirms this thinking; at least half of the patients and frequently far more are usually overweight.

A proper reducing cure consists not only of a low caloric diet; it must also include thyroid tablets, taken under strict medical supervision, and saline laxatives taken to reduce the weight (about 3 pounds a week) and to cleanse the whole system of just those waste products that cause the arthritis.

A reducing cure alone may often remove the symptoms of arthritis. It is usually advisable, however, to combine it with draining of the skin, as described earlier.

A few characteristic case histories will help to illustrate my recommendations:

Case 9. A sixty-year-old woman who had given birth to seven children had been suffering for more than three years from an allegedly steadily "progressive, degenerative" arthritis of both knees. All forms of the usual physical therapy, rest, heat, diathermy, massage, baths in hot springs, had been tried in vain. Even special clinics for arthritis had not been able to help. The patient could no longer walk by herself, needed the help of a companion and a cane.

In 1940, she was referred to me for treatment. I observed that both knees and calves, down to the ankles, looked like a single, swollen, cylindrical mass. The woman weighed one hundred sixty-five pounds, much too much for her very short stature five feet, one and a half inches. She also had, as so many of these patients do, a high blood pressure (185/95) and was extremely full-blooded. Strangely enough, nobody until then had suggested a reducing cure. Overspecialization often prevents the recognition of important general factors.

I prescribed a reducing treatment by which the patient lost thirty-six pounds within three months. Blistering plasters and artificial rashes were also applied on her legs in a very cautious way.

After treatment for five weeks, the patient was able to walk six to ten blocks every day without any help. After treatment for three months, she was capable of walking long distances without any distress whatsoever. Her well-being continued as long as

I followed her case, a period of five years. During this time, she was following my advice of keeping her weight down.

A few years later, I heard from mutual acquaintances that she had again neglected her weight, that nobody had taken care of her high blood pressure or of her plethora (fullness of blood), and that she had died of a stroke (cerebral hemorrhage). I believe that this could probably have been prevented by proper medical care and a repetition of her reducing cure.

Another story illustrates the futility of visiting health resorts for arthritis cures without taking into consideration the contributing factor of overweight.

Case 10. I met Mr. and Mrs. G. when I was traveling, more than twenty years ago, to the well-known warm springs resort, Bad Gastein, near Salzburg. They were fellow passengers in my railway compartment. Both were middle-aged and strikingly fat. It was not long before they began a conversation with me. Year after year, they told me, they traveled to Gastein, to get rid of their arthritis and rheumatism.

But they ate, I noticed, constantly. Not only did they report punctually for all their meals in the dining car but, in the intervals, they ate sandwiches, cake, chocolate, candy, and fruit. Grotesquely enough, these orgies of gluttony were regularly accompanied by the intake of aspirin, Atophan, and other antirheumatic drugs. At the rate they were going, they would probably need to make their pilgrimage to Gastein until the end of their lives.

The *importance of reducing* in overweight arthritis patients cannot be overemphasized. The following case history proves the point again:

Case 11. A fifty-five-year-old woman had been suffering since her menopause from "destructive" arthritis of both knees, combined with considerable swelling and immobility. At a special clinic for arthritis, spondylosis (arthritis of the spine) was also diagnosed. Following the trend of the times, her tonsils had been removed and all her teeth extracted. The operations had effected no improvement in her arthritis, however.

About fifteen years ago, she came under my care. She was unusually fat, weighing one hundred eighty-two pounds with a height of only five feet and two inches. As is often the case in such patients, she was also full-blooded with purple discoloration of the skin, bulging superficial veins, etc.

Characteristically, she had also gone through an operation for gallstones, and she suffered from renal colic (kidney stones), a general condition which corresponds to uric acid, or gouty diathesis. All this is the result of overloading of the metabolism and of the blood with surplus waste products. Nobody until then had suggested a reducing cure or other methods of cleansing the system of these harmful waste products.

I prescribed a reducing cure by which the patient lost thirty-two pounds within ten weeks. I also performed, at intervals, a number of very moderate bloodlettings (venesections) of the arm. On the painful spots, I applied blistering plasters and artificial rashes.

Before my treatment, the patient was able to walk at most two blocks and this only with great pain and with the help of a cane. After ten weeks of treatment, she was capable of walking one to two miles without any discomfort at all. She was so active and alert that nobody could imagine she had been declared a hopeless, incurable invalid only a few months ago.

This patient was presented by me, together with a number of other similar cases at a medical meeting in New York (1943) as examples of arthritic patients whom my methods had completely freed from complaints.

She was still completely free from complaints when, a year and a half later, she moved out of New York. Away from my observation and my advice, she neglected her diet and again put on weight. With the return of obesity, the arthritic complaints also came back. It was like an experiment of nature itself, proving the connection between arthritis and metabolic disturbances, particularly as they occur in conditions of overweight.

Another very significant case occurred in Vienna in 1935.

Case 12. A fifty-seven-year-old woman had been suffering since her menopause from polyarthritis, involving several joints. The knees, hips, and the spine were diseased; during the last year, her right arm had also become involved, particularly the elbow, the wrist, and fingers.

She had been treated in one of the most famous clinics of Europe, the Surgical University Clinic of Professor Baron Eiselsberg (my own teacher), in Vienna. She was given the usual therapy consisting of heat, massage, and aspirin and was finally discharged as unimproved with a splint of plaster cast reaching from the shoulder down to the finger tips. She complained of permanent pain. In desperation, she had begun to take morphine and other narcotics.

When the patient came under my care, I saw first of all that she was greatly overweight. Characteristically, also, she was dark-haired. Dark-haired people seem to have a more concentrated blood than light-haired individuals and therefore manifest a greater tendency to the formation of such deposits as gallstones, kidney stones, and those of arthritis just as a very concentrated solution of sugar or salt forms crystals or sediments much more easily than a diluted solution. This patient had already undergone a gallstone operation a few years previously. Her blood pressure at the time I saw her was 170/95.

I prescribed a reducing cure, making her weight go down twenty pounds in seven weeks. I applied artificial rashes and blistering plasters on the painful spots repeatedly. After two months, the patient was able to do all her household work; after three months, she could use her fingers well enough to play the piano again.

Just how decisive such a simple procedure can be, how it can affect the economic life, even change the whole future of a human being, the following case history will demonstrate:

Case 13. A fifty-eight-year-old business woman had already resigned herself to giving up her shop and to retiring to a home for the aged. During the last two years she had been almost unable to do any work because of the serious arthritic condition of her shoulders, knees, and hip. Her blood pressure was high H200/100. This combination of symptoms often found in arthritis points to the close relationship of the two conditions. More recently, the patient had been confined to bed because of phlebitis (inflammation of the veins) of both legs. Itching over the whole body also occurred, a condition that also indicated the presence of irritant metabolic waste products in the system. The patient was also overweight. Treatment with heat and aspirin had done nothing to alleviate her condition.

I prescribed a reducing cure and went on with methods to "clean" the system—sweating, purging, and bloodletting. Her weight came down from one hundred sixty-four to one hundred forty-six pounds in six weeks. By that time, all rheumatic pains as well as the phlebitis and the agonizing itching of the skin had disappeared. The woman gave up her plan of retirement and gladly went back to her business.

It is the overconcentration of modern specialists that often causes them to neglect such significant evidence as overweight and fullness of blood. Again and again, it must be stated that the patient should be observed as an entity, as a whole, and treatment accordingly given.

Questionable methods used in reducing

Many more persons in the United States are afraid of gaining weight today than in previous centuries. Slenderizing methods are common talk. Usually, these refer to diets. Milk farms for reducing purposes, very popular a few years ago, are still one of the favorite reducing procedures. People go there for days, even for weeks at a time, to live exclusively on milk. But milk, good as it may be for the suckling, disagrees with many adults. It can create flabbiness, gas, a surplus of acid, constipation, and weakness and dilatation of the stomach. It may coddle and weaken not only the stomach but also the whole body. "You are what you eat," and soft food makes you soft and sluggish. Therefore, the idea of reducing by an exclusive milk diet cannot be recommended.

The physicians of the Middle Ages and, later on, Paracelsus and, still later, English, French, and German physicians of the nineteenth century, noted also that the intake of a surplus of milk and milk products makes the blood so sticky and gelatinous that it increases a tendency to arthritis; this kind of food was forbidden to patients suffering from arthritis. In other words, "health food" is not always healthy.

Other individuals try to reduce through a *vegetarian* diet, a *raw diet,* or by living on *fruit juices* only. All these procedures upset the normal digestion and, in the long run, weaken the entire system.

Some try to kill the appetite by smoking large numbers of cigarettes or cigars, but this damages not only the circulation but also the nerves. There is such a thing as tobacco neuritis; even tobacco blindness can be incurred with damage to the optical nerve. Later I shall quote several examples to show how heavy smoking, very often, directly creates arthritis, neuralgia, and even palsy.

Recommended method for reducing

The reducing cure suggested by this author consists of 3 parts:

A low caloric diet

This means, insofar as is possible, no starchy food, no fats, and no sugar. It is relatively easy to take saccharine instead of sugar, and also to get along without fat. But I do not suggest mineral oil on salads as many do; mineral oil or liquid petrolatum upsets the function of the stomach, and is among those substances that may ultimately create cancer. Mineral oil is not recommended as a laxative for the same reasons.

The avoidance of starchy foods or the matter of providing substitutes for them may be difficult for some persons. The most practical way is to use foods similar to those used by diabetics, for example, protein bread, also called gluten bread. There are also other substitutes of farinaceous foods, such as special spaghetti, macaroni, crackers, and pastries, in which starch is replaced by protein. These products can be bought in most health food stores.*

The principal nutrition in a reducing cure should consist of meat in moderate amounts, eggs, fish and other seafood, cheese, vegetables, and fruit, the last not too sweet.

Potatoes and rice should be taken only in moderate amounts, if necessary. The usual cereals are out of the question.

As for drinking—plain water, carbonated water, eventually light wine mixed with seltzer, may be allowed in moderate amounts. Tea with lemon and saccharine may be recommended. A great help in reducing cures is good strong coffee of the best quality, particularly to be taken in the morning to prevent the initial weakness and fatigue that may originate from the withdrawal of such energy foods as sugar, starch, and fat.

Thyroid tablets

Two grains, twice a day, under strict medical supervision, are recommended whether the metabolism is below normal or not. Thyroid tablets help to burn up the surplus fat. At the same time they act, like their main ingredient, iodine, as a resolvent agent on all deposits, such as fat and arthritic deposits.

Saline laxatives

The best of these is Glauber's salt (sodium sulfate), which is the principal ingredient of many laxative mineral waters in Carlsbad and other famous health resorts. To make it more potable, this salt is mixed with an effervescent powder. The average dose for an adult is one heaping tablespoonful in half a pint of water before breakfast. This drug has various advantages. It accelerates the passage of food through the bowels, thus preventing full utilization of the food, a considerable help in reducing. It prevents, too,

Health food stores carry a wide variety of important natural foods which cannot be obtained in the usual food stores.

in hypersensitive individuals, possible autointoxication from the thyroid tablets. It also acts as a resolvent upon the fat and the arthritic deposits.

Long observation has shown, however, that cures based only on reducing diets never have the same beneficial effects in arthritis cases as the combined external and internal methods I have described. The reasons have been discussed in previous sections.

Fasting cures in arthritis

Fames totum corpus purgat—"Starvation cleans the whole system," said Galen, who wrote twenty volumes on medicine in the second century A.D. from which we can still learn.

Even today, particularly in Europe and especially in Germany, there are physicians specializing in fasting cures who have their own private clinics. They have achieved good results in some forms of arthritis. But such a fasting cure, lasting three weeks and by no means a pleasant procedure, must be carried out under strict and constant medical supervision. To me, it seems to be justified only in those conditions where no other method of healing is effective. I know of scarcely any such disease, except possibly certain forms of cancer that are too advanced to be operated on or radiated.

Another form of "hunger-and-thirst-cure" is the *Schroth treatment* in the former Austrio-Silesian village of Lindewiese, now a part of Czechoslovakia.

It was about a hundred years ago that the simple coachman Schroth, began his drastic starvation cure in his own sanitarium. It seemed to accomplish incredibly good results, particularly in certain chronic diseases that did not respond to the usual treatment. Stubborn skin diseases, neglected inveterate syphilis, and most important, crippling arthritis were rapidly improved or cured. This Schroth cure, which later became world-famous, lasted as a rule three weeks only. The patient was fed two stale white rolls and a cup of prune juice daily. Not even water was allowed. This was both a "hunger-and-thirst-cure." During the day, patients were allowed to walk around in the park of the sanitarium and in its wooded surroundings. For the night, each patient was wrapped in lukewarm sheets, topped by heavy blankets. This caused a strong elimination through the skin, a specific effect that apparently could not be produced through other methods. In severe cases, a very strong perspiration with a highly unpleasant odor was the result. On Sundays, every patient received one quart of a light white wine, to be consumed over the whole day. The wine-drinking on Sunday had a peculiarly stimulating effect, not only on the patient's mood but also on the eliminatory functions of the body. Actually, the results achieved by Schroth with thousands of cases over a period of many years were startlingly good.

Two examples from my own experience illustrate this method further:

Case 14. A sixty-year-old widow had been complaining since her menopause about increasing symptoms of chronic arthritis. Her knees, hips, spine, shoulders, and ankles were swollen and were becoming increasingly stiffened. She was also very much overweight. I was not too eager to treat this patient. Her fingers had also become involved, a localization that usually indicates a doubtful prognosis.

At that time, the Schroth cure was very much in vogue. The patient thought she might like to try it. I agreed. After three weeks, she wrote that her condition had improved so much that she could take walks lasting two hours every day; she had hardly been able to walk on the street at all before. She several times repeated this cure once a year and remained well as long as I could observe her.

Case 15. Another case concerns a patient whose history I have discussed earlier. She was the wife of the Austrian Minister of Commerce who was completely freed from her polyarthritis (involvement of her fingers, knees, shoulders, and ankles) by the secret herb potion of the lay healer in Graz. Several years later, as she approached the age of the menopause, the old symptoms of arthritis reappeared. She, too, had heard from her friends about the amazing results of the Schroth cure. Just as in the previous case, the fact that the fingers were involved prompted me to consent to her taking the Schroth cure. She remained in treatment for five weeks, came back completely free from pain, swelling, or stiffness. She, too, repeated the cure twice, three weeks each time, during the following two years, and then remained permanently well.

10 The function of the stomach, the liver and the gallbladder

Ancient wisdom has divided the human body into three stories or floors: the ground floor is the abdomen. It deals with solid and fluid matter, digesting our food, then producing and eliminating the waste products. The abdomen may therefore rightly be called the chemical laboratory of the body. As such, it is also the principal spot in which the products causing arthritis are manufactured.

The second floor, to continue this comparison, is the chest, which deals with more refined matter, with gas in the form of air, with its oxygen, nitrogen, and carbon dioxide compounds.

The third floor, finally, is the head with the organs of sense that deal with the waves of sound and light and with the electric waves of the brain.

Although all these functions are closely interrelated, the functions of the abdomen are of greatest concern to those who wish to understand and to treat successfully arthritis and its allied conditions. The function of the stomach, the bowels, the liver, and the kidneys may all contribute to the creation and cure of arthritis. From a practical viewpoint, the function of the stomach and of the liver are most important, and I shall discuss them in that order.

Stomach indigestion as a cause of arthritis

It was known in the days of Antiquity that disturbances of the stomach could cause or aggravate all kinds of diseases in most of the different organs. Today, we are all familiar with the fact that an acutely or chronically upset stomach may cause headache, dizziness, weakness, nervousness, palpitations of the heart, skin diseases, and all kinds of feverish conditions. The most frequent disease of the stomach, hyperacidity with its consequent indigestion, and largely accompanied by constipation, may increase the acidity in all tissues of the body and therefore also promote the production of uric acid, which is the most likely cause of arthritis.

In my own long experience, I have observed that those arthritis patients who are not overweight but rather strikingly thin are usually suffering from a causative condition of chronic indigestion.

It is an alarming fact that although chronic indigestion affects one out of every four or five residents in large cities, thus making it one of the most frequent of the chronic diseases today, it is not getting the attention or treatment it needs from modern laboratory medicine. On the contrary, the figures and laboratory tests referring to, for example, the acid content of the stomach or the length of time certain foodstuffs remain in the stomach, have too often been misleading. By that I mean that the laboratory figures may be exact but they are not related as they should be to a practically successful treatment.

To illustrate: Tests with the stomach tube have found that olive oil prevents the formation of acid in the stomach; but everyone knows that oil and other greasy foods are "heavy" foods, producing an unpleasant feeling. On the other hand, strong black coffee, according to laboratory tests, is supposed to promote the formation of acid; but, actually, it is felt in a beneficial way as a stimulant bitter tonic by the patient who suffers from a weak stomach. Finally, meat remains as long as six hours in the stomach; but meat is really very well tolerated because it binds the surplus acid. "The best food is roast meat" read the prescriptions of our practical earlier physicians.

No physician today, not even a specialized authority in the field, can cure an arthritic patient if he does not take into account the presence of a chronically upset stomach and its significance for arthritis.

Later, a diet for chronic indigestion is described in greater detail. In addition to the diet, bitter tonic remedies must be prescribed in order to counteract stomach weakness. It is not enough to neutralize the hyperacidity with alkalizers and to give belladonna for the pain. The bitter tonics are the real and radical remedies for indigestion. Such drugs are the preparations of gentian, vermouth, condurango, cinchona, and many other extracts of bitter herbs, therefore called stomach bitters.

One of the greatest and most frequent mistakes in the treatment of chronic indigestion is the prescription of milk. Usually one glass with every meal is prescribed; sometimes even a diet consisting exclusively of milk, cream, and cereals is advised. The effect of milk is to relax and weaken the stomach even more. Such patients can go on suffering for months and years without results. A tonifying diet should replace the milk diet.

Sour milk, buttermilk, or yogurt is very wholesome as food for patients suffering from chronic indigestion. Milk, of course, can be used for cooking purposes.

All this may sound "queer" or "revolutionary"! But practical experience confirms me. And all the earlier medical texts are of the same opinion.

Among meats, the best for a weak stomach are roast chicken, veal, and beef. Lamb and pork are harder to digest. Smoked boiled ham is easily digestible.

A sensitive stomach does not easily digest fresh fruits, vegetables, or salads, at least not at the beginning, not until the organ has become strengthened to the point that a balanced mixed diet can be recommended.

The type of food I have been discussing, if properly and individually prescribed, also prevents the formation of ulcers. The usual present-day treatment of indigestion or ulcer with milk and cream is, in my opinion, inadequate. I recommend a protein diet. In advanced cases of ulcer, six to ten raw eggs may be given as the only food that is well tolerated. After a few days, soft-boiled eggs with toast and boiled rice may be given. Very soon, ham and chicken may be added. More details for the attending physician can be found in my scientific *Textbook of Constitutional-Therapy.*

It may seem peculiar to discuss in such detail the diet and medication for chronic indigestion in a book on arthritis, but the high frequency of stomach trouble and its close relationship to the causes of arthritis justify such a diversion.

There are still a few other misunderstandings that need clarification. It is often suggested, even by physicians, that drinking six to eight glasses of water daily will help to "rinse" the body. This may be well tolerated by a healthy stomach but, in a weak stomach, such water intake increases acid formation, flabbiness, and dilatation. Moderate amounts of carbonated water, on the other hand, are an appetizing stimulant for the stomach, promoting eliminatory movements.

Outline of a diet for chronic indigestion

Again, considering the frequency of chronic indigestion in arthritis patients, I shall give a few hints that have proved beneficial in thousands of cases over a long period of years.

BREAKFAST

The best is strong black coffee, French roasted, of the very best quality. Sugar may be added, but no milk or cream.

One should take this black coffee on an empty stomach and give it five to ten minutes' time to work. It strengthens the stomach not only because of its caffeine content but also because it acts as a bitter and aromatic tonic. It creates appetite and empties the stomach downward. With many persons it results in a bowel movement through a kind of reflex action (gastro-colic reflex).

After a time, one or two soft-boiled eggs with toast and butter may be taken.

The usual fruit juices, particularly on an empty stomach, are not recommended. They create in a weak stomach acidity and heartburn. They are not so necessary a source of vitamins as modern advertising indicates. Any regular, mixed diet, including vegetables, salads, and fruit, provides sufficient vitamins. If desired and tolerated by the stomach, fruit juices may be taken at the end of the meal. Cereals are also not advisable for they slow down the digestion.

LUNCH

The simplest and best lunch consists of one or two sandwiches on toast, fresh rolls, or fresh sour rye bread, made with ham or other tender meat. If there is a desire to drink something, one may take carbonated water, tea with lemon and sugar, sour milk, yogurt, or good black coffee.

DINNER

Those who like soups may have strong beef soup or chicken soup with noodles, rice, or similar farinaceous products in it.

The principal dish should be meat of good quality, tender and well prepared. The fear of fried meat is not justified, if one uses good cooking fat such as butter, lard, chicken fat, or goose fat. Frying brings out the special flavor of meat better than broiling or boiling. It agrees particularly well with a hyperacid sensitive stomach.

Fish, as a substitute for meat, is not recommended for the weak stomach. It is more greasy and experience has shown that it is harder for many persons to digest than meat. When the digestive power of the stomach has improved, fish may be given, but also in a tasty form, moderately spiced. Spicing is important because it helps to stimulate and to support the digestive powers. Even heavier food is easier to digest if it is well spiced. The saltless and spiceless diet so widely recommended today is not good for a weak stomach.

The best supplement for meat is boiled rice. It is easier to digest than all other forms of starchy food.

Potatoes were originally called the "bread of the poor." Large amounts create a bloated belly with flatulence (gas) and therefore often disagree with a sensitive stomach. They may be taken in small amounts when the digestion has improved.

Vegetables in large quantities are not necessary. They may be useful as a vitamin source and as a necessary bulk for bowel movements. Among the vegetables, string beans, green peas, carrots, asparagus, turnips, red or white beets, and squash are recommended. They are more easily digested than cabbage, broccoli, spinach, and other vegetables.

As for salads, dense heads of lettuce are easily digestible. Tomatoes in a raw state are harder to digest than in steamed form or in a sauce. Cucumber salad is very heavy and does not suit a sensitive stomach. Mild soft pickles can be recommended.

Desserts are a problem for many. A greater concentration on farinaceous foods will help. Farinaceous foods in great variety can be made from the same dough as noodles. They may be prepared with tasty ingredients such as poppy seeds, nuts, marmalade, sweetened white cheese, etc. Fluffy pancakes are also easy to digest. Spaghetti and macaroni come next as a recommendation but the quality in noodles is better. Farinaceous foods, including pastry of all kinds, deserve more attention than they are getting in this country. European nations have learned that such foods add to the pleasure of eating, are easily digestible, and do not burden the metabolism as much as vegetables, fruits, or a surplus of meat. To help overcome the relative monotony of American desserts, European cookbooks may be consulted. Viennese cooking, a conglomeration of the cuisines of many nations—German, Hungarian, Italian, Bohemian, Croatian, Serbian, Polish, all part of the Austro-Hungarian monarchy at one time—may rank as the healthiest, being both appetizing and comparatively easy to digest.

Cheese is often recommended as a source of protein. It must be kept in mind, however, that spicy cheeses such as Roquefort, Camembert, bleu, and similar sharp and strong-smelling varieties, are more appetizing and therefore easier to digest than the bland white cheeses.

Fruits are a pleasant supplement in a balanced diet. For the person with a sensitive stomach certain fruits are preferable, either fresh or stewed or even as they are available in cans. The best for easy digestion are peaches, apricots, pears, pineapples, and bananas. On the other hand, apples, also apple sauce, prunes, oranges, and grapefuit very often create acid in the stomach, and heartburn. Grapefruit are better than oranges because of the bitterness, which is favorable for a sensitive stomach.

Among the fruit juices, only raspberry syrup and grape juice and, sometimes, sweet apple cider are well tolerated in a hyperacid condition. Among the vegetable juices, tomato juice, slightly spiced, as in tomato cocktail, agrees best with a sensitive stomach. Other vegetable juices frequently provoke gas pains and heartburn. The following case history is an ironic example of this type of reaction.

Case 15. Last year, I treated a thirty-five-year-old woman who was a beautician. Part of her complexion treatment consisted of advising her clients to live on a raw vegetable diet with plenty of fruit juices as a supplement. She became so convinced by her own salesmanship techniques that she decided to try the diet herself. Then she came to ask me what was wrong with her intestines. She had unbearably severe cramps in her bowels. I prescribed a reasonable mixed diet. The "unbearable" intestinal disease disappeared.

The tonic diet I have been describing must be adjusted to the individual taste and to the degree of the stomach disease. With improvement in the digestive powers of the stomach, the transition to a normal, balanced diet is gradually worked out.

How important, how indispensable even, the correction of a chronically upset stomach can be in the cure of arthritis may be illustrated by the following case. It is only one example among many similar ones.

Case 16.   In 1944, I saw a forty-seven-year-old housewife who had been suffering from polyarthritis for nine years. The shoulders, elbows, wrists, and ankles were involved. The fingers were disfigured and partly stiffened. The disease had become aggravated two years before with the onset of the patient's rather early menopause.

The condition was originally diagnosed as rheumatoid arthritis; the tonsils and teeth were removed in accordance with the recommendations of the time. There had been no improvement.

She had also had the usual treatment: diathermy, other forms of heat, and various injections, including gold. Large amounts of vitamin D tablets supplemented this treatment, also without success.

By the end of 1944, her condition had deteriorated so much that she was completely confined to her home.

It was at this point that I had the opportunity to examine the patient. She was emaciated, with a flabby, enormously dilated stomach, in which splashing noises could be produced, even six hours after the last fluid intake, a symptom very characteristic of sluggish digestion. The stomach had also dropped considerably (enteroptosis), reaching down far below the navel into the pelvis. In connection with this weakness of the stomach, stubborn constipation had manifested itself. In addition, the invisible perspiration of the skin was insufficient; the patient was unable to perspire even on hot summer days. This inability also contributes considerably to the retention of harmful and irritant metabolic waste products and therefore to the origin of arthritis and rheumatism.

I prescribed bitter tonics for the stomach and the tonic diet described earlier. Carefully chosen laxatives (e.g., tincture of aloes) were given to strengthen both the stomach and the whole body and to cleanse the system of accumulated harmful metabolic products. Aloe has been known as an ingredient in remedies for arthritis for many centuries. Sweating procedures and artificial rashes were applied. Progress was very slow. The case was a very advanced one, and had been judged practically hopeless by some of the previous doctors.

But within three months of my treatment, the patient was able to do all her own house work and her shopping. She was capable of walking long distances, even of dancing at a party.

When she decided to visit Saratoga Springs, the New York health resort she had been frequenting for cures during the past nine years, the nurses were amazed by the improvement she had made since the previous year.

Such a case history, typical, as I have said, of many others, again proves how important it is to treat not the diseased joints only or the arthritic condition only or even to hunt for alleged foci of infection and then to recommend extraction of tonsils or teeth. The essential point is to understand and to correct the individual's general condition, in this case the chronic indigestion, constipation, and inadequacy of skin perspiration of the patient.

Diseases of the liver and gallbladder as causative factors in arthritis

In cases of arthritic patients, we find strikingly often histories of gallbladder pain, caused by inflammation or gallstones, and even of surgical gallbladder removal. Recent statistics of the American Rheumatism Association disclose that between 30 and 50 per cent of all rheumatic patients have some kind of disturbance in the liver or gallbladder.

This is by no means a mere coincidence. Earlier physicians stated after long observation that disturbances of the blood, the lymph, and of the bile were among the most frequent causes of disease. Humoral pathology classified human temperaments according to differences in these fluids.

A surplus of *sangus,* Latin for blood, was supposed to characterize the vigorous and easily changing sanguine temperament.

A preponderance of phlegm or lymph was supposed to produce the quieter, more even phlegmatic temperament, also called the "lymphatic constitution."

A surplus of bile (in Greek *chole*), identified chemically as yellow bile, may involve the whole body. It was considered a characteristic of the energetic or choleric temperament. This disposition was particularly attributed to the men of action in history. Napoleon was, physically and mentally, a prominent example. Like all people of this type, he had a dark complexion. This was a basic theory about the temperaments—that highly energetic types were usually dark.

Ancient physicians also distinguished a second kind of bile, the black bile (in Greek *melancholia*), which was supposedly produced in the spleen. This hypothetical "black bile" could never be identified chemically. But the theory of the black bile has been a useful working hypothesis in explaining and in treating, more or less successfully, many symptoms that we classify today under the common heading of gouty or uric acid diathesis. The ancients called them "atrobiliary" (black bile) symptoms. To this group belong arthritis, melancholia, and cancer. If ever a remedy for cancer is found, it may very well consist of ridding the metabolism of waste products corresponding to the symptoms of black bile. The intuition of earlier physicians pointed to a close relationship between these symptoms and the cause of cancer. The black bile was believed to make the blood dark, thick, heavy, and acrid or sharp.

My own observations coincide with many of the earlier physicians. I have found that individuals with dark hair, eyes, and skin seem to have a more concentrated blood, charged with irritant metabolic products (probably caused by bile, as is the case with the dark coloration itself). These individuals therefore have a greater disposition to the severe forms of arthritis, such as "progressive" and "destructive" arthritis. This can be proved by statistics.

Consequently, arthritic dark-complexioned people are usually benefited by "blood thinning and blood purifying" remedies, such as saline laxatives and a large number of chemical drugs and herbs and also by a suitable bland diet.

The possibility that the coloration of a person may have a deep influence on his temperament and on his disposition to certain diseases is not as strange as it seems. The color of an object—a mineral, a chemical substance, a flower—gives definite hints about its chemical qualities. Roses of different colors have different scents. Egg yolks of brown eggs are more concentrated than those of white. Coloration in animals is accepted as an indicator of their temperament. The difference in the character of horses with black, white, brown, or rust coloration is well known. Among cattle, cows with white skin have a lesser resistance to tuberculosis than dark-colored cows. Human propensities for this disease are also different for light and dark individuals.

Purgation as a principal remedy for the cure of arthritis

Since arthritis is a metabolic disturbance, correction of the faulty metabolism, overcharged with irritant waste products, is of fundamental importance. The most effective way of cleaning the system has been and still is purging (with or without adequate dieting). Hence, the old medical axiom: *Qui bene purgat, bene curat*—"He who purges well (by bowel movements) cures well." This sentence represents one of the most important and elementary principles of practical medicine of all times and nations. Modern medicine, with its precariously unbalanced emphasis on laboratory research, has all but forgotten this principle, has all but forgotten, too, how many diseases can be cured by proper, skillful, and individualized purgation. Arthritis is one of these.

Galen, who has influenced scientific medicine for more than fifteen hundred years, reports that, in addition to many other diseases, he was able to cure the most advanced cases of arthritis by purgation only (sola purgatione), even patients who were so lame that they had to be brought to him "by cart and wagon."

During the centuries that followed Galen, numerous simple and compound drugs (herbs, minerals, and chemicals) were developed as more or less specific cures for arthritis. Many of them, by cleaning the system through specific purgatives, were effective in cases where we seem to be helpless today. A classic example of these are the Holy Bitters of the ancients, which with some variations were used successfully for the cure of arthritis up until a hundred years ago. In modern times, the French *Liqueur Laville* and the Italian *Pagliano Syrup* are among the best substitutes.

VOMITING IS OFTEN MOST EFFECTIVE IN STUBBORN CASES

Medicine is not a mere stumbling from one new discovery to the next by laboratory research. It is, more basically, the accumulated knowledge of the useful experience of earlier physicians, a vast body of knowledge that practicing medicine cannot afford to ignore. As I have said before, chronic diseases, arthritis among them, are medicine's Number One problem today. If earlier methods were more successful than our own, we have no choice but to examine those methods, to synthesize them with our own—in other words to do all we can toward the fulfilment of our medical purpose, which is to heal.

Earlier physicians distinguished two kinds of purgation, first, the purgation downward, by laxatives, and second, the purgation upward, by vomiting. To many modern ears, this may sound barbaric. But vomiting is a healing mechanism of nature itself! If a baby has taken in too much milk, he vomits it without any effort or distress. If we swallow harmful or upsetting substances, the stomach works to throw them up. Many infectious diseases start with vomiting, an indication to the physician that the harmful matter may have entered the system through the stomach. Our medical predecessors imitated this healing mechanism of nature by artificially induced vomiting. They developed it to a refined art, used it to accomplish many "miracle" cures in otherwise intractable cases.

Artificially induced vomiting can be achieved without causing too much discomfort if the physician knows how to do it. In arthritis, I had to use it very seldom—only in stubborn cases or if a quick cure for a localized pain (e.g. lumbago) was necessary. The following example is illustrative:

Case 17. A forty-year-old woman who held an important position in a large industrial concern in Vienna had been suffering for several weeks from a very painful lumbago and sciatica. She was confined to bed. The usual remedies—heat, aspirin, massage, liniments—had not helped. Even the artificial rash that I applied brought only partial relief, not the usual freedom from pain and stiffness it usually achieved. Since the patient had a very urgent business meeting scheduled for the same week, I prescribed an emetic.

On the very next day, the patient was completely free from pain, could move around freely. She continued well, was able to attend to her professional duties without any difficulty.

Numerous similar reports, concerning the often magiclike effects of emetics, can be found in the medical textbooks of the sixteenth, seventeenth, eighteenth, and early nineteenth centuries.

Case 18. The famous French surgeon of the seventeenth century, Ambroise Paré, was called to the Court of the King to treat a young nobleman. He had been suffering from a very stubborn and painful inflammation of the shoulder joint. His arm seemed almost to be paralyzed. Paré advised him to fill his stomach one evening with as much food and drink as he could take, and to follow this up the very next morning with a vomiting medicine. This was done. One day later, the patient could freely move his arm again. He suffered no more pain.

But why, one may ask, does vomiting have such a particularly healing effect on stubborn cases of arthritis and allied conditions? Vomiting stimulates to the utmost the center of the vegetative nervous system, the solar plexus, which controls the functioning of all our inner organs, particularly the stomach, the bowels, the liver, the heart, the lungs, the kidneys, the skin, the blood vessels, and most important, the lymphatic system. The last, if properly stimulated, promotes the mobilization and elimination of metabolic waste products. The solar plexus is also called the abdominal brain, as a counterpart of the brain in the head.

The significance of vomiting as a drastic but often lifesaving remedy was indicated by the famous Hufeland, one of the most successful physicians medicine has known. Hufeland considered vomiting, bloodletting, and opium as the three "heroes" or fundamental remedies of the medical art. These three procedures, as very few other remedies, may make the quick difference between life and death, or between a rapid cure and a long, protracted sickness. Vomiting may prevent, shorten, or mitigate many infectious diseases. Whooping cough is one example. Together with bloodletting (venesection), it was found to be lifesaving in edema of the lungs, in embolism (blood clot) of the pulmonary arteries, in dangerous attacks of bronchial asthma, and in many other critical or protracted conditions. Vomiting mostly provides quick and surprising cures in otherwise stubborn and lengthy asthma conditions among children.

In arthritis, vomiting, as I have explained, through its stimulating effect on the lymphatic system, enables the body to resolve exudations and deposits from painful or stiffened arthritic or rheumatic organs. When used, effective cures can usually be expected.

Sweating—a powerful remedy in arthritis and rheumatism

"One third of all diseases can be cured by sweating"—SYLVIUS, (famous seventeenth-century physician)

This famous statement, made by one of the greatest physicians in seventeenth-century Holland, can be understood if we realize that the skin is not only our largest organ, but also one of our most active organs of elimination. We usually forget that the skin discharges more than one pound of waste products every day through the so-called invisible perspiration, namely steam, carbon dioxide, and volatile fatty acids that produce the sour smell of sweat. The retention of the invisible perspiration has the toxic effect of self-poisoning. Blocking of this invisible perspiration by covering the skin with impermeable substances such as lacquer, often done for theatrical purposes, can be a dangerous procedure if the covering is not removed quickly. Suppression of this perspiration by extensive burns of the skin or by substances that close or tan the pores, such as gold paint or formaldehyde, for example, may if prolonged cause death within twenty-four hours.

Many individuals suffer from insufficient skin breathing, characterized by dry and rough skin and by an inability to sweat, even in hot weather. This is the case with many diabetics and also with arthritic patients.

It is an old experience that he who keeps his inner surface (the bowels) and his outer surface (the skin) very active is not likely to get sick.

Sweating has been developed through the ages as a powerful healing method. Humanity discovered very early the healing effect of sweating and ancient, even primitive nations had their steam baths in some form. Turkish, Russian, and Roman baths and the Finnish Sauna are, of course, well known. Remnants of the Roman baths can still be seen in their ruins as buildings of large and elaborate construction. Earlier cultures used steam baths much more regularly and frequently than we do. They systematically prevented and cured numerous diseases of middle and old age with them, particularly metabolic disturbances such as diabetes, arthritis, rheumatism, and allied conditions. We should revive both our interest and our understanding of the therapeutic value of these procedures today.

Hot baths alone are not enough. Steam baths are more effective. There are a number of steam baths in large cities, mostly patronized by middle-aged and elderly people. Visits to such baths are timeconsuming, however, and often rather expensive.

It seems more advisable for arthritis sufferers to have a sweating cabinet at home. In severe cases, treatments can then be taken several times a week, without leaving the house. There are different types and systems of sweating cabinets, constantly being modernized and improved. The best among them is a sweating cabinet heated by a small infrared heating apparatus that can be connected with any electric current in the house. The patient sits on the infrared heater, which is the size and shape of a kitchen stool. The patient and the heater are surrounded by a rollable wall of wooden wedges or shutters, covered on top by a waterproof closure through which the patient can put out his head. The shutters are lined with a material reflecting the infrared radiation. The whole cabinet may be rolled together like a carpet; it is light in weight, does not take much space, and can be put in any corner of the room.

Sweating is superior to other forms of heat (e.g. diathermy, short waves, etc.) because it promotes the elimination of waste products. If we keep in mind that arthritis is mainly a metabolic disturbance, resulting from overcharging of the system with certain irritant waste products, it is easy to understand why elimination through the bowels and through the skin is helpful.

Sweating, together with the other methods of treatment already discussed, helps to cure even the most stubborn cases of arthritis. A dramatic example is the following:

Case 19. A forty-five-year-old woman had been suffering from increasing pain of the whole back. This condition was diagnosed by experts and special clinics as an "incurable arthritis of the spine." Treatment had been given up as hopeless. The patient was a widow who had to support four children by working in a factory. She was made utterly desperate by the outlook of lifelong invalidism.

When I first saw her, she pleaded with me, "Is there no method and no doctor who can help me?"

My examination revealed insufficient breathing of the skin, characterized by the typical rough and dry skin quality. The patient admitted that she could not perspire, even in the summer. She was also overweight, a frequent combination with arthritis. I prescribed a reducing cure and daily sweating in a sweating cabinet. I also applied artificial rashes, bit by bit, over the whole spine.

Under this treatment, the complaints diminished rapidly. The "incurable" patient resumed her factory work after only four weeks of treatment.

11 Care of the skin in health and disease

A properly functioning skin protects the health by regulating the body temperature and by preventing and curing many diseases. Elimination through invisible perspiration and sweating, as I have described, are most essential. To help the reader at this point, I shall give a few hints about the care of the skin.

Cleaning of the skin by frequent, if possible daily bathing or showers must be considered first of all. Hot tub baths, often preferred in this country because they are so "relaxing," are not advised. They coddle the body and make it lazy and rather tired instead of hardening and tonifying it. The water should, at least, be cooled off by the end of the bath. Showers, beginning with luke warm and gradually getting colder, are much more stimulating.

Hydrotherapy has been elaborated into a highly specialized art.

It is used by modern naturopathic physicians and lay healers with great success. Among numerous systems that of the Catholic priest, Monsignor Kneipp, has become world-famous and is still practiced in special health resorts, particularly in Germany.

Air-bathing and *sun-bathing*, the latter in moderation, also contribute to the good functioning of the skin. In Antiquity, overweight patients were advised by their physicians to go about their daily work in half-undress, covered by a loin cloth only. Daily "rubbing" of the body was recommended in ancient Rome by Celsus for the purposes of preserving and recovering health. This was especially important for those leading a sedentary life.

Proper clothing is also very important. Many mistakes are made in this regard today, particularly by women. The old tightly laced corsets have been given up only to be replaced by tight elastic girdles, reaching from the lower part of the chest down to the thighs. Women tell themselves that this cannot be harmful because the material is "elastic." But these girdles not only hinder the invisible perspiration of the skin over a considerably large area but also strangle the liver, the diaphragm, the stomach, the kidneys, and the intestines of the abdomen, seriously interfering with their circulation. Many harmful consequences may be the result.

An illustration on this subject is the following case history:

Case 20. Some years ago, I treated a very good-looking English lady who had been suffering for a year and a half from violent lower backache and sciatica. She had consulted doctors in several of the best clinics but without getting any help. Finally, she was told by some orthopedic surgeon that only an operation, consisting of artifical stiffening of the lower spine, could help her.

When I examined her, I found that this patient, who was close to the menopause, was overweight with bulging breasts and hips. She also had a strikingly dry skin and was unable to perspire, even on hot summer days. As she undressed, I saw that she wore, in order to appear slender, an airtight corset of solid rubber, reaching from the armpits down to the middle of the thighs. Such an obstruction of the invisible perspiration can alone provoke rheumatic diseases by retention of harmful irritant metabolic waste products!

I prescribed a reducing cure, the daily use of a sweating cabinet, and induced artificial rashes over the whole painful area. Of course, she had to drop the corset at once.

Her condition improved rapidly. After five weeks, she was completely cured and remained so.

Counter-irritation or draining of the skin

Counter-irritation or draining of the skin is the most powerful healing method in arthritis and rheumatism; quicker and more surprisingly gratifying results are achieved than with any other method.

To free a suffering human being from agonizing pain is one of the highest and most important duties of the physician. The ancient classics expressed this fundamental principle with the sentence: Divinum opus est, dolorem tollere—It is a divine act to remove pain. A dedicated physician will move heaven and earth to fulfil this sacred duty, a duty that means much more than temporary soothing of the pain with sedatives or narcotics. True healing means removal of the deeper causes of the pain, permanently.

For arthritis, very few methods work in such a quick and permanent way as draining of the skin by vesication (blistering), by the creation of artificial rashes, or, in severe cases, of artificial sores, also called fontanellas, and in extremely·rare intractable cases, by the use of cauterization with the hot iron (under an anesthetic).

Labeling these methods as old-fashioned may be the blind spot of laboratory medicine. My own every-day experience and that of my associates over a period of more than forty years reveals the alarming fact that all over the world millions of people, stricken by arthritis, are suffering unnecessarily for months, for years, even for a lifetime. Why should simple and effective methods that were used successfully by the greatest masters among our medical predecessors and are being used successfully today be "labeled" and shoved aside? The attitude may almost be compared with religious, racial, or national fanaticism, which makes people impervious to the most obvious truths. With the pride of dogma, modern medicine claims to be the only way because it is founded on the laws of exact natural science—that is, mathematics, physics, and chemistry. But the advocates of this "exact" science overlook the important fact that even our best physical and chemical measurements are still too clumsy and inadequate to meet the complicated requirements of the living system and probably will always be that way. "Life begins where chemistry ends," said Liebig, one of the greatest nineteenth century scientists. I am both experienced and humble enough to agree with him.

Various degrees of counter-irritation

SKIN-REDDENING LINIMENTS AND PLASTERS

The mildest form of counter-irritation is the application of skin-reddening remedies such as the mustard plaster, liniment of ammonia, tincture of green soap, oil of chloroform, tincture of red pepper (capsicum), oil of wintergreen, camphorated alcohol, etc. Certain patent medicines are compounds of those ingredients, e.g., Pain Expeller, Sloan's Liniment, and many similar drugs. The early Red Indians successfully used petroleum or kerosene for compresses in painful rheumatic conditions. This is still effective today. It was used in the Army as effective emergency treatment for lumbago or sciatica. Compresses of benzine have a similar effect.

Turpentine was also used by earlier physicians as a liniment and for compresses. It is still worthwhile trying and often effective.

A number of artificial chemical substances, for example, methyl-salicylate, are used in rather high concentration as pain-soothing salves. The same principle in a very handy form has been put on the market under the name of Robugen, shaped like a lipstick (made in Esslingen, Germany).

How far away present-day understanding of counter-irritation is from reality may be gathered from the fact that mustard plasters, sold in the form of mustard papers the size of a post card, bear an inscription on the back that reads, "nonblistering"! This means that exactly the most effective action of mustard, namely blistering or draining of the skin, is anxiously evaded. The following story related to this subject sounds almost like a joke.

Case 21. A physician in California told me the following incident: He had prescribed such a mustard plaster for a woman suffering from violent lumbago and had told her to keep it on no longer than 15 minutes. The patient, completely exhausted from pain, found such relief through the plaster that she fell asleep for several hours. When she woke up, small blisters had formed and the backache had disappeared completely and permanently. The physician to whom she reported what happened, replied, "Were you lucky! I, myself, would never have dared to prescribe such a drastic cure for you."

Such superficial blisters heal in a few days by themselves and are therefore completely harmless.

VESICATION BY PLASTER OF SPANISH FLY

Earlier the origin and usage of this cantharides plaster is sufficiently described. I remember several cases of single swollen finger joints, especially the case of a young girl who was freed from pain and swelling by one single application of such a plaster. She exclaimed, "Oh, but this is like magic!" With that, she came nearer to the truth than many learned physicians of our time.

ARTIFICIAL SORES (ISSUES)

There are two kinds, a superficial sore and a deeper one; the latter is also called fontanella.

Superficial issues. It is an old surgical master trick, especially useful in arthritis of the hip joint, to create a superficial artificial sore on the great trochanter (the bulging part of the thigh bone, just below the hip joint). The procedure is the following: The physician applies a plaster of Spanish fly, about the size of two to four postage stamps, for twenty-four hours. When a blister has formed, the loose skin that covers the blister is removed with a piece of cotton. Afterward, the physician cauterizes the raw surface with concentrated nitric acid, slowly, step by step touching the raw wound with an applicator soaked in that acid. This causes a short burning sensation that disappears after one or two minutes. This can be done under local anesthesia to eliminate pain. In this way, a scab is formed over the whole blistered area, either on the same day or in successive sessions, if the patient is too sensitive for concentrated treatment. Very often, immediately after such a cauterization, the patients notice that the pain and stiffness in the joints have diminished considerably or even disappeared and that they can move freely again. This painting with acid has to be repeated about once a week for six weeks. It is hardly painful after the first cauterization. Patients learn to walk again, free from pain and without the crutches or canes that they formerly used.

An interesting example of the effectiveness of such an artificial sore in arthritis of the hip is the following case history:

Case 22. More than twenty years ago, I delivered a lecture to the Medical Society of Amsterdam, concerning the usefulness of earlier methods of healing. The day after the lecture, a family doctor brought to me one of his patients, a young married woman who, since the birth of her child two years earlier, had been having trouble with her hip joint. She suffered from a painful chronic inflammation (coxitis) and could walk only a few steps, supported by a cane. The usual treatment by the local specialists had not helped.

I applied a plaster of Spanish fly on the spot and cauterized it the following day with nitric acid. Immediately after the cauterization, the patient exclaimed: "Doctor, this is the first time in two years that I can move my hip joint without any pain." In fact, she walked around without limping and even succeeded in doing some of the gymnastic exercises she had enjoyed before she became ill. I advised the physician to keep the artificial sore open for six weeks (by cauterizing once a week). The patient remained permanently free from complaints. She visited me two years later in Vienna and presented herself as definitely cured.

This happened more than twenty years ago, but the procedure is equally effective today. With its use, I have avoided a number of surgical operations (complete stiffening of the joint), which had been suggested to such patients as their only possible help.

Fontanellas (deeper artificial sores) as a cure for stiffened joints. In contrast to the superficial sores described above, there is a similar method, particularly useful in stiffened joints (ankylosis), consisting of deeper issues in the skin.

The great surgeons of the eighteenth and early nineteenth century expressly said: "Great is the power of fontanellas; they even cure ankylosis."

This procedure, too, unfortunately is disregarded by most modern surgeons. They seem to prefer mechanical methods such as traction, stretching the joint in narcosis, and even operations. The fontanella method is carried out in the following way: A blistering plaster the size of a small coin (penny) is applied for twenty-four hours. Afterward, the physician cauterizes a small hole in the skin with a pencil of caustic potash. After a few days, the scab is shed and the remaining hole is filled with a dry irritant object, e.g., a glass pearl which, covered by a band aid, keeps the wound open for several weeks. There is a continuing trickle of small amounts of serum. Such wounds never become infected. This simple procedure loosens stiffened joints, and as these sores discharge fluid like a fountain, they are called fontanella. This method is particularly useful in cases of stiffening arthritis of the knee joint.

I first learned the amazing effect of this method in an unexpected way.

Case 23. At the beginning of my private practice in Vienna (1919), a middle-aged woman, a fruiterer from the market place, came into my office. She complained of the common symptoms of the menopause. But when I examined her, I found to my great surprise an artificial ulcer on her lower leg about the size of a quarter, which looked as if it had been punched out with a sharp iron instrument. When I asked her what this sore meant, she sneered, "Oh, all you learned doctors, you don't know anything! For years, I have this swollen, painful knee joint, almost completely stiff. I spent and spent money, going from one doctor to another. They did not help. It was the lay healer out of town who cured me. He has cured many such. He burnt this hole into my skin. Since that time, I can walk. And I walk without pain!" Further questions on my part revealed that the hole had been made with a cauterizing substance.

I did not learn anything of that kind during my training at the Surgical University Clinic. Surprised at this experience, I searched again in old medical textbooks and found this procedure as a regular part of "minor surgery" in earlier medical systems. Since that time, I have been using this "method" in numerous cases with great success.

I presented a number of such patients at a meeting of the Medical Society of Vienna in 1936. Among them was the following:

Case 24. The patient was an elderly woman who made a living by housecleaning. She was forced to give up her livelihood because one of her knees was greatly swollen, almost double the normal size, also painful and stiffened. Since she was overweight, I immediately prescribed a reducing cure. I also applied blistering plasters and finally a small fontanella. Her condition improved from week to week. After six weeks, she was so much better that she could resume her housecleaning job. She continued her reducing regime and remained permanently free from complaints.

12 *Should arthritic people smoke?*

Why do people smoke at all? Many enjoy smoking as a treat. Others use it as a stimulant; still others, as a kind of sedative, to relax. Moderate smoking may be harmless and add to the pleasures of life.

Exaggerated smoking, however, may be harmful, even dangerous for the health.

Very few smokers realize that exaggerated smoking may damage all organs of the body. The skin becomes dry and leathery and, with this the important invisible perspiration is diminished. Consequently, acid irritant metabolic products are retained in the body and may provoke or aggravate rheumatic diseases.

In women, excessive smoking may damage the ovaries, and the

menstruation becomes too scanty, which again produces a disposition to arthritis.

Some people smoke in order to numb the appetite and thus prevent putting on weight. But they are also producing a weakening of the digestive organs, such as the salivary glands, lymph glands, liver, stomach, pancreas, kidneys, and spleen.

Excess of nicotine may lead to heart diseases (e.g., angina pectoris), to hardening of the arteries with high blood pressure and vascular spasms (cramps of the blood vessels). Even some forms of cancer involving the lips, the tongue, the larynx, and the lungs may be caused by too much smoking.

Heavy cigarette smoking may provoke too—and this is a reaction not so widely known—the most serious forms of arthritis, neuritis, and neuralgia. The opticus nerve can occasionally be damaged so much that tobacco blindness occurs. Unfortunately, it is very difficult to persuade arthritis sufferers to cut down their smoking or, as is sometimes necessary, to give it up completely. The following case histories are examples of situations where excessive smoking was an important factor in the arthritic condition:

Case 25. A forty-six-year-old, otherwise robust-looking, handsome man came limping into my office. He explained that he had been suffering for a year and a half from increasing pain in the lower part of his spine and from violent sciatica of the left leg. The pain was intense. All possible usual treatments had failed. The once dapper, elegantly dressed gentleman now had to wear a heavy harnesslike corset made of steel and leather. A major operation, artificial stiffening of the lower spine, was being planned for him.

Not one of the numerous outstanding physicians whom the patient had consulted in France and in America had asked him about smoking. This question should be asked of every rheumatic or arthritic patient, just as the physician inquires about digestion, weight, perspiration, blood pressure, etc.

When I saw the patient, he admitted that he was a chain smoker, consuming between thirty and forty cigarettes a day. I finally persuaded him to stop smoking, prescribed a reducing cure and applied artificial rashes on the spine. The patient recovered completely within seven weeks. He has been completely well for more than eight years.

Case 26. A friend of the above patient's displayed almost the same morbid symptoms. He, too, was about forty-five years old and a heavy cigarette smoker. For two years, he had been complaining of increasing pain in the lower spine with irradiation into both legs. The usual treatment had failed.

Noted arthritis specialists had diagnosed arthritis of the spine complicated by a slipped disc and suggested the artificial stiffening of the spine operation. Until the operation could be scheduled, this man, too, had to wear the clumsy corset of steel and leather.

Nobody had advised him against smoking. He was not even asked about it although his clothes actually reeked from the thirty cigarettes a day he was consuming.

I made it a strict condition that he stop smoking. Since he, too, was a little overweight, I prescribed a reducing cure and applied artificial rashes. After the first treatment, he was able to do without his corset. Within a few weeks, he was free of all complaints. He remained so as long as he continued the hygienic way of life I had prescribed. The allegedly slipped disc no longer gave him any trouble. The original diagnosis about it was evidently incorrect.

Case 27. A forty-two-year-old bank teller had been suffering for several years from repeated attacks of arthritis of his right shoulder. The attacks usually lasted three or more weeks. The patient treated himself with the usual home remedies, heat and aspirin.

But this time, the attack had already lasted ten weeks. The patient was becoming incapacitated. He was in danger of losing his job.

By the time I was consulted, he could not move his arm at all, and had the condition often referred to as "frozen shoulder." He, too, admitted that he smoked two packs of cigarettes a day. I advised him that I would treat him only on the condition that he give up smoking completely while under treatment and that he smoke only with moderation afterwards.

I applied an artificial rash over the whole painful area. After one week, the rash dried up. The patient could move his arm freely without any pain. The fear and memory of the previous pain was strong enough to hold him to moderate smoking habits. He remained well during all the years I kept in contact with him.

Case 28. A publicly known case of "bursitis" or rather more correctly "arthritis of the shoulder" was that of President Eisenhower, a smoker accustomed for years to thirty to forty cigarettes a day. He had suffered for three years under the usual treatment. With my method, this kind of disease can be cured in three weeks.

Excessive smoking may be combined with overweight, high blood pressure, chronic indigestion, and insufficient perspiration or menstruation. All these irregularities must be corrected. The exaggerated smoking must cease if treatment is to give quick and lasting results.

Sometimes, instead of arthritis, polyneuritis, an involvement of many nerves, may occur. My former associate, Dr. Albert W. Bauer, formerly of Vienna, now in London, had such an experience:

Case 29. He was consulted by a forty-year-old man who complained of violent nerve pains in the whole body, with weakness and numbness of the limbs. Outstanding medical authorities diagnosed polyneuritis but could not help the patient.

Dr. Bauer was immediately startled by the intensive smell of cigarettes exuding from the patient. He learned that this man had been smoking thirty to forty cigarettes a day for seven years. Prohibition of smoking and the methods of elimination already noted restored the health of the patient within a few weeks.

13   *Review of current medical treatment*

Psychosomatic factors

It is fashionable today to speak of psychosomatic medicine. This is usually interpreted, however, from one point of view only: how mental strain influences the body in health and disease. The other side of the picture, how neurotic conditions and even mental diseases can be cured by treating the body, must also be considered. The latest methods used for some mental diseases, incidentally, have been giving the latter point of view greater emphasis recently.

Medical observation has long noted that worries, grief, constant rushing, hurry, and excitement may damage not only the nerves but also various functions of the body. Everyone knows that terror, fear, and anxiety may spoil the appetite. Most sufferers know that arguments during meals may produce gallstone attacks. In brief, unpleasant emotions may have a generally unfavorable influence on all organs. Particularly, it may produce a surplus of a faulty quality of the bile with transition into the blood and the metabolism. Arthritis and neuralgia, too, may be caused by this mechanism. Not in vain does the French proverb say, *Ne vous faites pas de mauvais sang*—"Do not corrupt your blood by excitement."

These are long established observations. It is only the slogan, "stress," that has been introduced as something original by Dr. Selye, who verified the well-known facts in the laboratory.

Arthritis, however, can never be cured by psychotherapy. Only the proper internal and external, general and local medication, described in the previous chapters, has proved to be an effective cure.

Value or uselessness of the usual methods of treatment

Most patients who come under my care have already tried all the usual official treatments. They come only because the treatments have not helped them. I may mention, too, that some years ago an editorial of the *Journal of the American Medical Association* stated expressly that all the usual treatments were useless. I shall now discuss the various common treatments briefly:

Rest

This is recommended by many arthritis specialists. I apply blistering, get the pain and stiffness to disappear, and encourage just the opposite, namely early, almost immediate active movement.

Physical therapy

This includes the application of the various forms of heat, radiation, and electricity. I have already stated that sweating is the most effective application of heat. The other forms, such as short waves or diathermy, have no worthwhile effect at all.

Massage

Valuable as massage may be in cases of stiffening after an injury, I do not advocate it in any form of arthritis. By increasing the irritation and inflammation, it may even prove to be harmful.

Chiropractic and osteopathy

These two methods are closely related, almost identical, actually, and separated only because of the rivalry of their founders. Both methods are based on the supposition that vibration, knocking, twisting, and similar manipulations on the vertebrae of the spine may have a wholesome reflectoric effect on the nerves that branch off from the various sections of the spine, and an accompanying effect on various other organs. This treatment, also called manipulation, may be useful in certain minor disorders of the spine or the back, e.g., in lumbago. But in arthritis of the spine and of other joints I have never seen successful results obtained through chiropractic or osteopathic treatment, although I have examined many patients who consulted chiropractors and osteopaths after ineffective treatment by current medical methods.

Radiation with X rays

Beneficial as X rays are for diagnostic purpose, their usefulness as a method of healing is greatly overestimated. Their application may even be dangerous.

I know of many specialists who use radiation with X rays as a routine treatment for arthritis of the shoulder. The pain may perhaps disappear but it has a tendency to return after a time, on the same spot or on other less favorable locations.

Our medical predecessors strictly warned us not to push gouty or arthritic matter back into the system, where it may settle in vital organs and cause great damage. They feared particularly that the heart and the lungs might be affected through such a procedure. Earlier medicine had no X rays. The old physicians knew enough, however, to refrain from applying repressive medication (e.g., preparations of lead) which, like X ray, can drive the gouty matter deeper into the system. What is needed, instead, is to create an escape for it through blistering and similar methods of elimination.

Today nobody, at least within my own knowledge, hesitates to treat arthritis with X rays, although closer observation proves the great damage that can be done. I have seen a number of cases in which a heart attack (angina pectoris or coronary thrombosis) occurred after X-ray treatment of arthritis of the shoulder. I would like to quote one such example now:

Case 30. A sixty-five-year-old man had been suffering for three years from arthritis of his right shoulder. All the usual treatments had been applied in vain, including numerous novocain injections that were considered, incidentally, even more horrible by the patient than the agonizing arthritic pain. Finally, he was treated by X ray and was stricken with a coronary thrombosis. The conclusion that the arthritic matter was pushed back from the joints to the heart by the X rays is obvious. We have observed the same in many similar cases. It was for this reason that earlier physicians called angina pectoris (including coronary thrombosis) a "gout attack" of the heart. The dangerous complication in the case quoted probably could have been avoided by treating the arthritis with methods of elimination.

X-ray treatment of arthritis should definitely be discouraged entirely.

Injections

Many drugs have been used, by injection, as a cure for arthritis. Most of them have not given satisfactory results. A number of specialists and hospitals once tried protein injections, in order to create an artificial fever. The results were unsatisfactory. The same holds true for injections of sulfur, iodine, and salicylates.

Then came the era of the so-called block therapy with novocain injections. These anesthetic injections were given directly on the painful spot, for example on the shoulder joint. In cases of sciatica, they tried to block the nerve supply of the sick organ. Two similar methods have been tried in Germany recently and are recommended by a number of physicians. They are the segment therapy and the impletol therapy. The first method blocks the pain in large areas or segments by injections at the root of the nerve, near the spine. The second method consists of injections of a mixture of novocain with caffeine into specific trigger points.

But all these injections are unfortunately only of transitory value. They do not correct the basic metabolic disturbance.

Injections of gold were introduced about ten years ago. The healing results are still uncertain. Harmful aftereffects, such as liver damage, hemorrhages into the skin, etc., have occurred in a number of cases.

The "wonder drugs," ACTH and cortisone with its derivatives, hydrocortisone and meticortone, given by mouth and by injections, seemed at first to be most successful. Cortisone and ACTH were intended for use only in rheumatoid arthritis, however, and this concerns only 5 to a maximum of 10 per cent of all arthritis cases. In the more common type of arthritis, osteoarthritis, ACTH and cortisone have no effect at all. These drugs have also produced so many harmful and dangerous side effects that they may be used only with the utmost caution.

Injections of formic acid and bee venom are also unreliable; whereas the sting of live bees is often successful.

Internal medication

Salicylates such as aspirin and its derivatives are most commonly prescribed for arthritis. Pyramidon and a similar product, Butazolidin, are also given, not only as a pain-soothing remedy but also with the hope of a cure.

I have explained earlier that certain herb extracts, e.g., that of Herba Gratiolae (herb of mercy), resins such as aloe, scammonium, etc., and finally the specific drug for gout, colchicine, are still used with success.

Most important is the use of mild preparations of mercury and antimony, both of which, by stimulating the lymphatic system, act as useful agents in combating chronic inflammations and metabolic disturbances. It was for this reason, as I have mentioned earlier, that mercury was called by earlier physicians the "tamer" or "conquerer" of arthritis. I have achieved some very good results by prescribing small amounts of calomel, the mildest preparation of mercury, given repeatedly over short periods of time with all the necessary precautions.

Orthopedic and surgical treatment

Orthopedic surgeons usually like to employ physical therapy and mechanical procedures, such as traction, as part of their treatment —particularly in arthritis of the spine or in cases of stiffened joints. Braces and splints are also widely recommended by orthopedic specialists. In conditions of arthritis of the spine, heavy corsets of steel and leather reaching from the armpits down to the middle of the thigh are prescribed, sometimes almost for life.

In all such cases, I succeeded in freeing the patient from pain and stiffness within a few weeks by the application of artificial rashes. Of course, proper general care, that is, reducing cures, correction of digestion, tobacco elimination, etc., as indicated by the individual case, was always a basic part of the treatment. But usually, after the first week of treatment, the corsets could be left off and never worn again.

Surgical interference in arthritis cases consists principally of so-called fusion operations, that is "bloody" stiffening of single joints, such as hips and knees, or of certain sections of the spine. After such operations, the patient must remain in a plaster cast for at least six to eight weeks, until the surgically treated parts have healed together.

Very often, such stiffening operations are performed in the lower part of the spine. But frequently, the arthritis begins to spread upward toward the chest and neck, in spite of the operation.

The fundamental cause of arthritis, it must be repeated again, is a metabolic disturbance such as chronic gout, which cannot be cured by mere mechanical interference. Such operations are therefore useless; they are sometimes also dangerous.

As one example out of my own experience, I wish to quote the following case history:

Case 31. A woman in her change of life had been treated by noted specialists for osteoarthritis of the lower spine and hip, but without success. She suffered severe pain, walked only with great effort, usually limped.

I had the opportunity to take over the treatment. A moderate reducing cure was prescribed for the overweight. Artificial rashes and plaster of Spanish fly were applied on the painful spots. After a treatment of six weeks, the patient was able to resume all her normal activities without any discomfort.

A few months later, she traveled to Switzerland for a summer vacation, wrote to me happily that she was playing golf every morning and making little trips into the mountains almost every afternoon.

Half a year after that, not having had any medical supervision, she suffered a slight relapse in connection with her menopause. This could have been remedied by a few treatments in a very short time.

Her husband, however, and some of her fashionable friends suggested that she should be cured thoroughly "once and for all" by an orthopedic operation. Without asking my advice she entered a hospital, and a major operation, consisting of stiffening of the lower spine, was performed.

Unfortunately, the wound did not heal. She had to stay in bed for several months, attended by day and night nurses. Finally, an infection of the spinal cord developed. The patient died in permanent distress six months after the operation.

Summarizing again, orthopedic operations in arthritis are necessary only in a small minority of selected cases. Stiffening of the spine is not only dangerous, but it does not stop the arthritic process, which may spread upward from the stiffened lower spine to the chest and the neck. Operations can never cure the metabolic disturbance which is the real cause of arthritis.

PART TWO

SPECIAL DISCUSSION

14 *Arthritis: summary*

Osteoarthritis, as I have pointed out, is by far the most frequent and therefore, practically speaking, the most dominant form of arthritis. Usually, it is a general or systemic disease, involving the whole body. When it is localized in one joint only, it is often due to injury or permanent strain.

It is not true, as is generally believed, that the cause of arthritis is still unknown and that there is no cure for it. We do know both the nature and the cause of arthritis. It is a metabolic disease, closely related to, if not identical with, uric acid diathesis or chronic gout.

Effective treatment of arthritis consists of removing the harmful irritant metabolic waste products in all possible ways. The most important forms of elimination or removal are:

1. *Draining of the skin* on the affected area by various forms of counter-irritation.
2. *Purging* through the bowels with specific antiarthritic remedies.
3. Intensive *sweating*.
4. *Bloodletting* in cases of high blood pressure or plethora (fullness of blood).
5. Using specific anti-inflammatory, antidyscrasic (blood-purifying) and *antiarthritic remedies,* such as recommended herbs and chemicals.

All this has been confirmed by this author and his associates over a period of more than forty years.

We must also remember that the most common form of arthritis, osteoarthritis, involving 90 to 95 per cent of all arthritis cases, attacks, for the most part, middle-aged or elderly people. Furthermore, the female sex is strikingly prevalent among the sufferers. The proportion is 4 to 1. Women after the menopause are the most frequent victims. Some of the recent popular books on arthritis have brought this knowledge to the public as a new discovery, a revelation. Actually, it is an old, old story in the earlier medical texts.

Very often, the question arises as to whether there is a specific diet for arthritis. The answer is "no." The diet must be chosen according to the general condition of the individual. Overweight people must reduce. A method is indicated earlier. Undernourished patients are usually found to be suffering from chronic indigestion. They must follow a diet that will cure the irregularities of the stomach. Individuals with an overcharged metabolism will be benefited by a blander diet with restrictions on meat, spices, and alcohol.

With the understanding and treatment I have recommended, the outlook for the cure of arthritis becomes much more optimistic. There remain hardly any intractable cases. Even such forms of arthritis as current medical thinking dismisses as "irresistibly progressive," arthritis of the spine, for example, can usually be arrested and freed from pain, stiffness, and other discomforts within a few weeks.

The "wonder drugs," ACTH, cortisone, or its derivatives do *not* work wonders for *osteorarthritis*. The same holds true for certain highly recommended local treatments, such as novocain injections and its different modifications. All these methods cannot correct the disturbed metabolism that is the deeper cause of osteoarthritis.

15 Special localizations of arthritis and rheumatism

I shall now describe the various locations in different joints and other organs that require certain modifications of the general and local methods of treatment.

◆

Arthritis of the shoulder

You may wake up one morning with a sudden pain in the shoulder joint and may be unable to move your arm at all. This *frozen shoulder* is one of the most frequent localizations of arthritis.

How constantly we need and use our arms we fully realize only when pain makes us no longer able to comb our hair, to wash ourselves, to shave, to dress, or to attend to any of our daily occupations. The "frozen shoulder" pain is often so violent that the slightest movement feels like agony and the arm seems paralyzed.

At first, the patient usually tries to treat himself with a heating pad and some pain-soothing drug, such as aspirin. The common medical treatment today consists of diathermy, massage, local injections of novocain, and radiation with X rays. I have stated that X-ray treatment may apparently remove a local pain but may have harmful consequences on other organs.

Proper treatment with my methods *cures every such case of arthritis of* the shoulder within one to three weeks.

Case 32. Not too long ago, I treated a fifty-year-old unmarried woman who, with the beginning of her menopause, began to suffer from a very painful arthritis of her right shoulder joint. As the housekeeper of a very high-ranking clergyman in New York, she had been treated by the best available specialists for six weeks with the usual methods. There had been no improvement.

The condition had most inaccurately been dismissed as "bursitis." Examination revealed that the whole joint was involved, that is, the capsule, the tendons, and the surrounding nerves and muscles.

In acute cases of short duration, my kind of treatment usually succeeds in a surprisingly short time. It was true in this case, too. Two plasters of Spanish fly were applied at an interval of five days, and small amounts of calomel (as an anti-inflammatory remedy) were prescribed. After ten days, the patient said she had no more complaints. She could move her arm in all directions without any discomfort. She suffered no relapse at any time during the following year of my observation.

Another very similar experience also took place recently.

Case 33. A fifty-eight-year-old physician practicing in New York had been suffering for five weeks from a very painful arthritis of his right shoulder. The pain radiated into the fingers and upward into the neck, so that the suspicion of *complicating radiculitis* (inflammation of the roots of the nerves near the spine) was justified. As the patient was about to leave for a vacation in Florida, I could see him only twice. Here, too, plaster of Spanish fly, and calomel given internally, brought about *a complete cure within a week*.

The following case is a more complicated one:

Case 34. A sixty-one-year-old former actress had been suffering from diabetes for a period of three years. She had also undergone a gallbladder operation two months earlier. In the middle of January, 1957, she complained of a violent and very painful arthritis of her right shoulder with neuralgic pain reaching into the fingers. The family doctor made the superficial diagnosis of "bursitis," apparently because in such cases small calcifications in the bursa (the mucous sac near the joint) can be seen on the X-ray picture. The whole joint was involved, however, and a second painful spot was situated in the middle of the upper arm. An artificial rash, gradually applied from the shoulder down to the wrist, and a plaster of Spanish fly on the particularly painful spot restored free movement and freedom from pain within three weeks. Small amounts of calomel were given by mouth to promote a quick cure. The patient remained well permanently.

The great difference in the duration of arthritis between the "official" treatment and my methods can again be illustrated by the following case:

Case 35. The patient was sixty years old. She had always had a tendency to obesity, but since her menopause at the age of forty-nine she had been gaining much more rapidly, and weighed two hundred fifty-six pounds. She complained of traveling rheumatic, neuralgic, and arthritic pains in the whole body. In 1944, the pain became concentrated in her left shoulder. A noted specialist in orthopedic surgery treated her in a large hospital for four months. First, he removed the bursa, by operation. When this did not bring the expected relief, he tried various injections—novocain, iodine, vaccines, bee venom, etc. No internal treatment, except for pain-soothing drugs, was given. Completely discouraged, the patient refused any further medical treatment and tried to get along with pain-soothing remedies only.

In January, 1945, she came to consult me. She complained of pain in the whole left shoulder joint, but also of neuralgia that radiated downward to the elbow. I applied an artificial rash over the painful area. In less than one week, the pain had disappeared completely. Of course, a reducing cure and other means to improve the metabolism and the heavily disturbed general condition were prescribed at the same time.

A condition that had not even shown improvement with the usual treatment of several months was cured within a week!

To those who must live by the work of their hands, the decision between lengthy and ineffective treatment and a practical method that works quickly and well is, naturally, of most vital importance, as the following case demonstrates:

Case 36. Mrs. A. M., a fifty-one-year-old laundress, was almost unable to work and therefore faced complete lack of subsistence. For four months, the pains in both her shoulder joints had been growing alarmingly worse. For more than a year, she had been attending a public clinic and getting the usual treatment of radiations with X rays, heat, massage, novocain injections, etc. It had not been able to prevent the progressive deterioration of her condition.

In January, 1943, the patient came under my care. Artificial rashes, alternating with plasters of Spanish fly on the painful shoulder joints, combined with proper internal antiarthritic treatment, such as saline laxatives, resin of guajac and calomel removed the pain and the stiffness completely within four weeks. After a treatment of six weeks, the patient was able to resume her work. She has remained well since that time.

Case 37. One of my most dramatic cases is the following: An otherwise robust and energetic woman, fifty-eight years old, had been suffering for more than eight months from increasing pain and stiffness of her left shoulder. Gradually, the pain reached from the upper arm and forearm down to the thumb. The generally used treatment did not help. The patient had sleepless nights, was resorting to the strongest sedatives, even morphine. Although she was not at all hypersensitive, on the contrary, had a great deal of strength and self-control, she was often forced to cry out with her pain. It was an excruciating pain because the nerve near the joint and supplying the thumb (the radialis nerve) was actively involved.

She was told by her physician that there was no quick cure and that the disease might still last a very long time. She came to me, in New York, after a train ride of seventeen hours from Chicago, in 1939.

Step by step, an artificial rash was applied over the whole painful area. From the very first, the pain diminished quickly and the mobility of the arm increased from day to day.

After a treatment of three days, pain-soothing remedies were no longer necessary. The same procedure was repeated three times at intervals of one week. Saline laxatives and sweating procdures were applied at the same time. At the end of three weeks, the patient returned home, free of complaints.

Three years later, she came back to New York with similar complaints in her hip and knee. Again, she was sent home after three weeks, free from pain. In the scientific edition of my book on arthritis, numerous such cases are described in detail.

Arthritis of the elbow, the wrists, and the fingers

Arthritis of the elbow

An isolated osteoarthritis of the elbow occurs relatively seldom but it, too, can be cured quickly through the methods described in this book. An interesting case that came to my attention a few years ago is this one:

Case 38. A sixteen-year-old, otherwise healthy girl had been complaining for three years about increasing pain, stiffness, and swelling in her left elbow. She had consulted noted specialists and hospitals in New York, was told that she would have to wait until she was twenty-one years old (until the end of her growing period), and that then an operation would be performed. In the meantime, nothing could be prescribed but heat applications.

The patient worked as a telephone operator and complained of pain at each movement, especially when lifting objects, even the extremely light attachments of the telephone switchboard. Letting the arm hang down and taking a position in bed were also painful.

In February, 1951, I took over the treatment. The X-ray picture showed nothing for only the capsule of the joint was diseased, and not the bones. I applied an artificial rash. Two days later, she came into the office feeling better already. She could straighten out her arm in the elbow joint to a considerable degree.

After a treatment of ten days, with the artificial rash repeated twice, she was able to go back to work.

After the third week of treatment, she was able to straighten out the arm completely. In one more week, the pain was completely gone and treatment could be interrupted. The patient came once a month for a check-up over the period of a year. No relapse occurred. The recovery was permanent. Blistering or counter-irritation had been successful in this case of arthritis of the "soft parts," too, where modern methods had been helpless.

Arthritis of the wrist

Arthritis of the wrist also seldom occurs alone. It is more often a part of a generalized arthritis. Sometimes, however, especially in cases where the wrist has been strained, the isolated condition occurs. The case of the Tirolean tailor mentioned previously is an example. His arthritis of the wrist was cured within one week by a single application of a blistering plaster.

Another example is the following:

Case 39. A fifty-six-year-old lithographer, straining his right wrist constantly in the performance of his work, had been sick for about a year. His wrist was painfully swollen; he was afraid he would be unable to work much longer. A few years earlier, he had been suffering from a rheumatic lower backache. I had cured that very quickly through artificial rashes and internal medication, the latter for the overcharged metabolism. This time, I used plaster of Spanish fly. The pain disappeared in less than a week. At the same time, I treated his general condition, a kind of "chronic gout," with remedies to cleanse the entire system.

Arthritis of the wrist, if it is not of a tuberculous nature, may be cured in an amazingly short time by draining of the skin, probably because the joint is so flat and the draining of harmful products through the skin is so much easier here than elsewhere.

Arthritis of the fingers

In contrast, arthritis of the fingers is one of the most difficult conditions for a physician to cure. It seems that those forms of arthritis that involve the small joints are both much more resistant to treatment and more firmly rooted in a deeper underlying cause. One may, nevertheless, succeed in improving or even curing this condition by very careful attention to the individual disturbances of the metabolism. Counter-irritation, intensive sweating procedures, and anti-inflammatory specific remedies, particularly small amounts of calomel, may help to bring about a successful cure.

Arthritis of the fingers attacks not only elderly people in the form of osteoarthritis, but frequently also younger women with insufficient menstruation and inadequate perspiration. These cases more often belong to the rheumatoid type of arthritis.

Arthritis of the fingers, as part of a generalized polyarthritis, is demonstrated by the following examples:

Case 40. A forty-eight-year-old secretary had stopped menstruating two years earlier. Premature menopause, natural or artificial, usually creates a greater disposition to polyarthritis. Her hips, knees, ankles, lower jaw, shoulders, elbows, and fingers had been involved during the last few years. The fingers had become so painful, swollen, and stiffened that she was barely able to use her typewriter. All the usual methods of treatment, even bee venom and Vitamin D, had not helped.

I found an extremely dry skin, learned that the patient could not perspire even on hot days. For this, I prescribed a sweating box and internal sweat-producing remedies. Locally, I applied various forms of blistering, also gave small amounts of calomel. Within six weeks, the condition had improved so much that the patient was able to type again, gradually up to eight hours a day without any difficulty. The whole treatment was continued for several months. She remained permanently well.

Those cases in which only single fingers are swollen are much simpler to handle. Often, one or two plasters of Spanish fly are enough to accomplish a cure.

Not to be confused with the arthritis of the finger joints are the deposits of calcium near the finger tips, in women after change of life. These swellings are called Heberden's nodes. They are usually not painful but cannot be removed except by surgery.

The so-called intractable cases of arthritis of the fingers can definitely be improved a great deal. The physician must take into account, in both diagnosis and treatment, the general causative factors, such as overweight, fullness of blood, overcharging of the metabolism by uric acid, and insufficient perspiration and menstruation.

In those cases where cortisone has been prescribed and has not helped, preparations of metallic substances such as mercury and antimony, given by mouth, often have a more positive specific effect. These are powerful remedies, well known to our earlier physicians who began to use them in the sixteenth century. The idea of using them more extensively today needs to be seriously considered by modern arthritis specialists.

Arthritis of the knee joint

Painful swelling and stiffness of the knee joint occur almost more often than arthritis of the shoulder, especially in women after the menopause. Walking, getting up, sitting down, bending, and going upstairs are difficult, often impossible. Here, too, currently popular treatment usually fails, and such cases are pessimistically disposed of as "irresistibly progressive," "destructive," and "incurable."

But even in arthritis of the knee joint, blistering with plaster of

Spanish fly, artificial rashes and, if necessary, fontanellas together with proper general care can radically change the outlook. Improvement sets in quickly, continues from week to week, and usually, within four to eight weeks, makes possible free movement, without much distress. Reducing cures, particularly, often bring about a remarkable change for the better, not only by relieving the weight-bearing joints but also through the general effect of dispersing inflammation, swelling, and stiffness.

When I was lecturing at medical Congresses in Germany last summer, I heard a fellow lecturer, a very well-known naturopathic physician, dismiss cases of arthritis of the knee joints as "degenerative" and "destructive" and state flatly that it was very difficult to arrest such cases, much less cure them. Even with regular care, he said, with strict diet, massage, and physical therapy, it would take at least one to two years before some improvement could be seen. This naturopathic physician did not mention in his treatment the draining of the skin, which experience has proved a more effective method for the treatment of knee-joint arthritis than all the methods he mentioned. Some examples follow:

Case 41. Mrs. J. M., fifty-nine years old, was suffering for two years from osteoarthritis of the right knee. The usual treatment with short waves, ultraviolet radiation, and injections did not help. Finally, one of her attending physicians advised her, "Don't waste your money; arthritis is incurable." Modern medicine had once again ignored the obvious: the general condition, the significant symptoms, the relationship of both to indicated treatment. The patient was overweight. I prescribed a reducing cure. The symptomatology indicated local irritant waste deposits. I applied an artificial rash on the painful spot once a week. The condition improved so rapidly that after three weeks the patient was able to walk long distances. The swelling of the knee was visibly reduced. After a treatment of only six weeks, Mrs. J. M. was discharged without any complaints.

Case 42. Mrs. H. S., fifty-eight years old, had undergone a hysterectomy at the age of thirty-eight. During the last eleven years, she had been suffering from arthritis, rheumatism, and neuralgic pains that traveled around in the whole body, a complex of symptoms often seen after artificial menopause. There was increasing stiffness in all joints and also occasional attacks of trigeminal (facial) neuralgia. The skin of the patient was dry; she seldom perspired and then only with difficulty. Buzzing in both ears revealed similar morbid processes in those organs.

The main complaint of the patient was pain and cracking in both knee joints. She could walk only with great pain and enormous effort. The usual treatment with hormones (for the artificial menopause) and physiotherapy had effected no improvement.

In June, 1943, the patient came under my care. I concentrated the general treatment on various means of improving the metabolism. Specific laxatives and frequent use of a sweating cabinet were prescribed. Repeated applications of plasters of Spanish fly on both knees were made. Within six weeks, the condition was improved so much that the patient was able to walk as long and as far as she wanted with no pain and no effort. This patient was presented at a medical meeting in New York together with other similar cases.

The necessity of individualized general treatment besides the local therapy of the diseased joint can also be gathered from the following history:

Case 43. Mrs. G. C., fifty-seven years old, short in stature, weighing one hundred ninety-one pounds, with intensely red skin (indicating a surplus of blood), and large varicose veins on the legs, came to me for treatment. "Destructive arthritis" of both knees, especially on the right side, was the pessimistic official diagnosis. Considerable swelling, deformation, and pain at the slightest movement were evident. The patient was hardly able to walk more than one block and even that, only when supported by a cane. She had been unsuccessfully treated in several clinics with protein injections, bee venom, short waves, and X rays.

I began treatment with a reducing cure, brought her weight down four pounds a week. Twice a week, I put plasters of Spanish fly on the most painful spots. After three weeks, the condition was so much better that the patient was able to walk a mile a day. The reducing cure was continued. The patient had no relapse during the follow-up period of four years.

Case 44. A sixty-eight-year-old Catholic mission priest, accustomed to traveling long distances in the course of his occupation, had been suffering for three years from increasing swelling, pain, and stiffening of both knees. He could now walk only short distances with great effort and, though supported by a cane, he limped severely. All the usual treatments did not help.

I took over the treatment about nine years ago. I combined a reducing cure with blistering once a week, alternating on both knees. In two months, I restored the health of the patient so completely that he was entirely free of difficulty and was able to make his taxing journeys across the American continent and even to accept arduous assignments in Europe. Despite his advancing age, he has remained consistently well.

Another striking example that proves the difference in results between so many of the "official" treatments and the method I recommend is the following:

Case 45. A fifty-nine-year-old woman living in upstate New York was intending to sell her chicken farm and to retire from work. She had been suffering for six years from "progressive" arthritis in both knees with disfiguring swelling, stiffening, and great pain.

She had spent large amounts of money, consulted the most famous arthritis specialists. Nobody gave her any hope for improvement. In the usual manner, the disease was considered degenerative and irresistibly progressive. No thought was given to the idea that arthritis, like chronic gout, may form deposits that can be removed.

It was easy to see that the woman was both much too heavy and full-blooded. Her blood vessels were visibly overfilled. I prescribed an energetic reducing cure, performed several bloodlettings (venesections) and applied intensive draining of the skin on both knees. After only three weeks, she had lost twenty-two pounds and the mobility of the knees was back to normal.

With instructions to continue her reducing cure, she returned to her farm, again able to attend to her work. This change in treatment was, of course, decisive for the whole future of her family.

Such things ocur in my clinical and private practice almost every day.

◆

Arthritis of the hip joint (coxitis)

Arthritis of the hip joint may occur even in very young children or in teenagers. Then it is almost always tuberculosis of the joint. Modern treatment, consisting of plaster casts, rest, and radiation with sunlight, may take years and its outcome is uncertain. Faster and better results were achieved by the earlier physicians and, also recently, by me, with a treatment combining skin draining and the internal use of mild preparations of mercury and antimony. In recent years some good and encouraging results in tuberculosis of the joints were obtained by modern antibiotics such as streptomycin.

Case 46. Among several similar cases, I remember a schoolteacher, a woman of about forty, who was living in Eisenstadt, not far from Vienna. She had been treated for several years for a chronic tuberculous inflammation of the hip joint at the famous orthopedic University Clinic of Professor Adolf Lorenz in Vienna. Plaster cast and rest were the only remedies given to her. After a time, she was able to move about and to go back to work but, from time to time, she suffered severe attacks of pain that confined her to her home.

During one such attack, the lady came to me for advice. I applied a plaster of Spanish fly on the painful spot and prescribed small amounts of calomel to combat the inflammation. In a few days, the pain diminished considerably, and finally disappeared completely. This treatment had to be repeated, but only for a few days once or twice a year. The patient was able to work at her profession without any difficulty and without the frequent painful interruptions she had suffered before.

Another form of chronic inflammation of the hip joint occurs as a consequence of congenital displacement (luxation) of the hip joint. This occurs only in women. Timely operative correction of the condition is one of the highlights of modern orthopedic surgery. But in later years, osteoarthritis may develop in such joints as a consequence of strain. I have freed such patients from pain repeatedly, also by counter-irritation.

The common arthritis of the hip joint usually develops only in middle-aged or elderly people. In women, it often bears a close relationship to the menopause.

Such patients complain of pain, restriction of mobility, stiffening, and finally increasing difficulties in walking. According to present day concepts, this condition is a destructive or degenerative, deforming arthritis for which there is no cure except rest, plaster cast, and finally an operation, performed either by stiffening of the joint through fusion of both ends or by replacing the head of the femur (thigh bone) with a metallic substitute.

Such drastic action is usually unnecessary. It is possible in many if not in all cases to restore the free mobility and freedom from pain by counter-irritation and proper general care. Reducing cures in overweight people often have a dramatic effect, but the application of artificial rashes, blisters, and particularly of a superficial sore on the bulging part of the thigh bone (great trochanter) in such cases are of the utmost importance. Very often stories of such cures, as, for example, the woman from Amsterdam who walked after a single treatment, seem to be magic, "miracle cures." They are neither magic nor miracles. They are based on medical theories and methods that can be used by every physician who understands them. I would like to quote a few more such cases:

Case 47.   The wife of a high-ranking official of the University of Vienna, a woman approaching the years of her menopause, became fat, suffered from mental depression, acnelike eruptions of the skin, neuralgia, and chronic arthritis of her spine, neck, and wrists. Finally, also, her right hip joint became so painful that she could move only with difficulty.

She had tried all the usual treatments, even a fasting cure, but without any success. All of this was in the early 1930's. Then, too, fashionable "official" medicine was neglecting the practical methods. But the lady decided to consult me. I applied a superficial sore on the bulging part of the hip joint and prescribed a reducing cure. The pain disappeared quickly and permanently from the hip joint. Gradually also, the other symptoms of arthritis vanished. The patient was capable of taking long walks, of performing the gymnastic exercises in which she was interested, and even of resuming her mountain-hiking excursions on Sundays.

Another example concerns osteoarthritis developed after the fracture of the hip joint, as often happens in such injuries:

Case 48. A sixty-year-old woman suffered a fracture of the neck of the hip joint. An operation was performed by one of the best surgeons of the Johns Hopkins University in Baltimore. He used the excellent method of inserting a long nail between the two ends of the fracture. In spite of the fact that the fracture healed perfectly in a correct position, a so-called traumatic arthritis of the hip joint developed. The patient could walk only with the use of two crutches, and even then with great pain.

Even this outstanding surgical clinic knew of no procedure that could relieve the pain and stiffness of the hip joint.

In this condition, eight years ago, the patient came to New York and consulted me. Her overweight and the fact that she was a constant smoker had been overlooked. I prescribed a reducing cure, insisted that she stop smoking completely, and applied alternating vesication with plaster of Spanish fly, artificial rashes, and an artificial sore on the bulging part of the joint.

The condition improved rapidly. In three weeks, she could give up the crutches. She was supported only slightly by a cane, was able to walk, and even to dance. The previously completely discouraged patient felt, in her own words, "newborn."

This, too, is not an isolated, unusual case. Such surprising results occur very often in my clinical and private practice. As I said, they can be accomplished by any physician who knows the methods of counter-irritation and also takes into account the proper general care needed for special cases, in this case obesity and exaggerated smoking.

Case 49. A sixty-one-year-old woman whom I had successfully treated many years ago for osteoarthritis of both knee joints began to suffer in 1951 from an arthritis of her left hip joint. The pain was violent and she could walk only a few steps with great effort. After applying home remedies for several days without any relief, she came again to me for medical care.

I applied on the outer part of the hip joint an artificial sore, the size of four postage stamps. The patient was able to walk immediately. By the next day, she said she had no more pain. The sore spot was kept open for six weeks. The patient has never suffered pain again. She is completely cured.

Case 50. In a village near the city of Salzburg, a sixty-two-year-old woman had been suffering for six years from a very painful arthritis of the left hip joint. On the basis of X-ray pictures, the diagnosis of "destructive arthritis" was made. All kinds of injections and other treatments, even health resorts, had been tried in vain. The patient had to use crutches, could walk only short, agonizing distances. Finally, she was declared an incurable case.

In March, 1933, she came to Vienna and was referred to me. Characteristically, she had gone through a gallbladder operation seven years earlier. She was dark-haired with an olive complexion, thus belonging to the "biliary" type which, in itself, as I have discussed previously, has an increased disposition to severe arthritis. Moreover, she was overweight with a very high blood pressure.

No attempt had been made until then to bring down her weight. I prescribed a reducing cure immediately. I also applied, right at the start, an artificial sore on the hip joint, and began the establishment of artificial rashes.

In three weeks, the patient was able to throw away her crutches and, soon afterwards, also her cane. In three months, she wrote me that she was walking a whole hour from her village to the nearest church on Sundays.

A check-up four years later proved that the hip joint was still freely movable and painless. This patient, together with similar cases, was presented for demonstration purposes at the Medical Society in Vienna, in 1933.

The following case history is also an important one:

Case 51. A forty-four-year-old woman, an official of the Motor Vehicle Bureau of the City of New York, had undergone, at the age of thirty-nine, a hysterectomy which, as I have explained, often creates an increased disposition to severe arthritis. This patient fell ill in October, 1950, complaining of a very painful chronic inflammation of her hip joint.

Treatment by the family doctor and afterward at one of the most important orthopedic clinics of New York had consisted of heat, aspirin, penicillin, and even cortisone, although in such a case of osteoarthritis, this drug is not effective at all. No relief was obtained. The patient was confined to bed for two months. She was finally told her X-ray pictures showed "progressive destructive arthritis." She would probably never be able to walk in a normal way. It would take a very long time to help her achieve even partial movement.

In February, 1951, I took over the treatment. The patient had to be carried into my office by two companions. I applied an artificial sore on the hip, which I kept open for two months. I also covered the whole painful area outside of the artificial sore with an artificial rash that I kept going for several weeks.

After a treatment of six weeks, the patient was able to walk several blocks by herself.

From week to week, pain and stiffness diminished. After a treatment of three months, she was able to walk normally and could go back to her job.

I presented this case, as well as other similar cases, at a medical meeting of the Stuyvesant Polyclinic in May, 1951. It is now more than six years later. The patient is still well.

Case 52. Quite a similar story concerns a fifty-year-old headwaiter who had been suffering for two and a half years from increasing pain and stiffness in his right hip joint.

When the usual orthopedic treatment did not bring him any relief, he went to a chiropractor. This treatment lasted several months but did not help either.

In October, 1950, I began to treat him. Since the patient was very much overweight, I prescribed a reducing cure; I also advised him to stop smoking the short pipe he kept in his mouth all through the day. I applied an artificial sore on the hip joint, kept it open for two months. One week after the beginning of treatment, I added an artificial rash over the whole painful area of the hip joint. The patient came for treatment only once a week.

Two weeks after the start of treatment, the patient was able to bend his knees and squat without difficulty. Four weeks after the beginning of treatment, he could walk long distances without a cane and also perform various kinds of gymnastic exercises. He thought he was ready to stop treatment. I advised him to continue the counter-irritation of the skin treatments for another short period. The reducing cure also needed to be continued.

After a total treatment of two months, he lost thirty-two pounds. He did not limp any longer, had no more pain, was able to walk almost indefinitely.

The patient and his relatives called it a "miracle." All previously consulted physicians had told him: "We do not know the cause of arthritis. Therefore, a cure is impossible." Both medical reason and the large number of accumulated facts point to the contrary, prove that such cures are definitely possible.

Arthritis of the feet and the toes

Acute gout occurs almost exclusively in men and has its characteristic location in the big toe.

The common chronic, mostly noninfectious arthritis may also attack the other toes, the ankle bones, and the middle foot.

Very often, one can find arthritis that is caused by an inflamed flat foot. This is a sad condition, particularly frequent in women. Vanity and high-pressure advertising seem to have combined in bringing about a situation where about 95 per cent of all women have crippled feet. Heels that are too high and soles that are too narrow can destroy the arch of the foot early in life. The flat foot results. The weight of the body, which should rest on the basic joint of the big toe, the small toe, and the heel, now rests on the fore-end of the bones of the middle foot and on the toes. The latter are often squeezed together, losing their original round shape, becoming crippled, often clawlike, twisted, and covered with corns and calluses.

The pain that such conditions cause may sometimes reach from the foot higher up through the whole leg. If there is special disposition, arthritis of the toes and of the ankle joint may also develop. Good comfortable shoes, and in the case of definite arthritis, counter-irritation of the skin and proper general care may effect quick improvement and cure of such painful feet.

In America, the deformation of the feet has gone so far that a new medical specialty, that of chiropody or podiatry has originated. And orthopedic surgeons, instead of correcting the twisted joint of the big toe, sometimes just "let it go" by recommending the surgical removal of bunions.

Borderline cases between chronic gout and chronic arthritis of the toes and ankle joint occur particularly often in men, after the age of forty. Overweight and heavy smoking are often contributing factors. Removal of these general causes and proper counter-irritation of the skin can often cure such patients in a few days or weeks even when they have already been incapacitated for many months.

Case 53. In the summer of 1950, a fifty-two-year-old owner of a bake shop came to my office in a desperate mood. He could not put his foot down because of a violent pain in his right heel and around the ankle joint. He was unable to work. The usual treatment—diathermy, aspirin, injections—applied for five weeks, had not helped.

The patient was suffering from an inflamed flat foot with inflammation of the tendon sheets and, according to the X-ray pictures, also from arthritic deposits on the bones of the middle foot and the ankle joints.

I prescribed a necessary reducing cure, restricted his exaggerated smoking, and applied a strong artificial rash over the whole painful area. The rash dried up within five days, the pain disappeared, and the patient could return to his work.

Cases 54 and 55. Similar conditions prevailed in two other male patients, a taxi driver and a headwaiter in a bar, both middle-aged men. They had been suffering for several months from painful swelling of the ankle joints. One of these patients also complained of pain in the knee joint.

All the usual treatments had been tried, had not succeeded. Both patients had been unable to work for several months.

As soon as I took over the treatment, I prescribed a reducing cure for both overweight patients and applied counter-irritation of the skin. They were freed from pain within three weeks and able to work again. They had no relapse.

All this looks very simple. One might even say that it was self-evident. To earlier medicine, it was just that. Current research, focusing on the new, however, has neglected the old, has almost forgotten it. But this is only a stage in medical history. When the novelty has worn off, so to speak, our research scientists will turn their considerable talents, I am sure, to a reinvestigation of the theories and principles I am reviewing. Their confirmation will lead to the more precise diagnoses and the more practical healing methods the treatment of chronic diseases so urgently demands.

Arthritis of the spine

(including lower backache)

Backaches in general, and even more often, lower backaches of various kinds are very frequent, the latter especially often in women. There are manifold causes for this condition, among them anemia, general weakness, weakness of the muscles of the back, muscle weakness combined with bad posture, etc. But diseases of the inner organs, of the chest, the abdomen, (liver, kidney), and the pelvis, particularly enteroptosis (dropped bowels and stomach) may also cause lower backache. One of the most common causes is flabbiness, dilatation, and dropping of the stomach, combined with indigestion and constipation.

In the pelvic region, hemorrhoids, diseases of the bladder, and of the prostate gland in men may cause lower backache, too. In women, inflammation or displacement of the genital organs and tumors may also be causes of lower backache.

Therefore in each case of persistent pain in the lower back, a thorough medical examination must take place. I remember one such patient, treated for a rheumatic ailment of his lower spine who was actually suffering from cancer of the intestines.

Sudden lower backache, called lumbago, often combined with sciatic pain, will be discussed in a later paragraph.

I want to discuss now arthritis of the spine, a condition where both the bones and the ligaments may become painful and stiffened. Strangely enough, arthritis of the spine has been separated medically from the other arthritic diseases and considered as a separate condition. The result has been to give the impression of quite a peculiar and isolated morbid disease. Some authorities have even gone so far as to declare that arthritis of the spine is a particularly malignant, irresistibly progressive condition that inevitably leads to permanent invalidism. The belief is also current that arthritis of the spine belongs principally to the unfavorable "rheumatoid" form of arthritis. These are false concepts. It is because of these false concepts that the outlook of a cure for arthritis of the spine is still generally a gloomy one. I will demonstrate that *such an outlook is not at all justified*.

Each nation, depending on its own medical research workers, has called arthritis of the spine by a different name. The Russians call it Bechterew's disease, the French, Pierre-Marie's, the English, Paget's, and the Germans, Struempell's disease. This is unnecessary confusion that upsets the proper judgment and treatment of this ailment.

Much better results can be attained if one considers arthritis of the spine just a partial location of generalized arthritis, usually of osteoarthritis; most such patients have arthritic complaints in other joints at the same time.

There is only one relatively rare, unfavorable form of arthritis of the spine that occurs almost exclusively in young men for still unknown causes. For the time being, very little can be done to help those patients.

On the other hand, more than 95 per cent of all cases of arthritis of the spine belong to the harmless group of noninfectious osteoarthritis, which, I have pointed out repeatedly, must be understood as a metabolic disturbance, similar to chronic gout. As such, it can be greatly improved or cured in most cases in the relatively short time of several weeks.

It is partly the general routine of current treatment that has caused such a pessimistic feeling about a cure for arthritis of the spine. Rest, application of heat, pain-soothing internal and external remedies, radiations, massage, bathing cures, orthopedic machines for traction and stretching, plaster casts, harnesslike corsets of steel and leather, reaching from the neck to the thighs —all these treatments are useless. But proper general care and counter-irritation on the painful spots usually bring about an amazingly quick improvement and a lasting cure.

I have already described four such cases in previous chapters; I can add many hundreds of others. Fortunately real bony stiffening bridges between the single bones of the spine occur very seldom, and then only in neglected cases. The common form of arthritis of the spine (just as in the case of the other joints) involves much more often the surrounding soft parts (capsules, ligaments, or tendons) by formation of painful deposits. Such conditions of the soft parts can be remedied by the same methods as used for other joints.

In recent years, as a new complication, the idea of the "slipped discs" have been introduced. Some surgeons have tried to remove these protruding soft parts by a major operation. Other experts have found, however, that more conservative methods can be used. I shall describe these in a following chapter.

One can categorize arthritis of the spine, according to its different sections, into arthritis of the neck, the chest, the lumbar region, and that of the sacral and coccyx bones.

Arthritis of the spine of the neck

Usually again, middle-aged or elderly people, particularly women, are affected. Such patients complain of cracking and pain with each movement. Turning and bending of the neck become difficult, making dressing, eating, and drinking painful labors. Also in bed, these patients find it difficult to get into a comfortable position.

The usual treatment rarely succeeds and patients are commonly fitted with braces of plaster cast or leather, reaching down from the chin to the shoulders.

Since the nerves that supply the shoulder joints and the arms leave the spinal cord between the seven vertebrae of the neck, we often find pains irradiating into the arms, down to the fingers. This condition is also called "radiculitis," which means inflammation of the spinal roots of the nerves.

Case 56. Only recently, I started to treat a sixty-year-old man whose arthritis of the neck had begun nine years ago. All movements of the neck were painful to him. The treatment he had been receiving helped the pain in the neck area to subside gradually but neuritis of both arms down to the fingertips remained. The patient could not use his hands for writing or dressing himself, felt "almost paralyzed," and was utterly discouraged. Had he been treated at the very start of his disease by intensive counter-irritation of the neck, all these neuralgic and paralyzing conditions in his arms and hands would not have occurred.

I began a very careful general treatment, consisting of small amounts of calomel, alternating with the antiarthritic French remedy, Liqueur Laville. At the same time, counter-irritation was applied, step by step, on all painful spots. The condition improved steadily from week to week. By now, the worst of the agonizing pain is over, though treatment must still be continued.

In some of these cases, treatment must be repeated from time to time for a few days. Usually, I succeed in achieving permanent freedom from complaints in the initial treatment of a few weeks only.

Case 57. A fifty-six-year-old woman, the wife of a landowner in Canada, came to New York to consult me. She had the history of an artificial menopause, induced by an operation performed when she was forty-eight. Numerous observations have indicated that premature artificial menopause creates a particular disposition to arthritis of the spine. For the past year and a half she had been suffering from increasing pain and very disagreeable cracking of the spine of the neck. The pains also radiated into both shoulders and into the occiput (back of the head). All possible medical authorities had been consulted and all common methods of treatment had been tried (injections of novocain, vaccines, hormones, vitamins, radiation with X ray, etc.). Even osteopathic treatment had been undertaken but without success.

I applied an artificial rash over the whole painful area, three times, at weekly intervals. Internally, I prescribed small amounts of calomel, alternating with tartaric salts. After three weeks, the pain had disappeared completely. Only the sensation of cracking remained. As the patient had to return to Canada, I advised her to continue proper internal medication and to apply, externally, certain irritant liniments (e.g., Richter's Pain Expeller).

Four months later, she came to New York for a check-up examination. She told me she was completely free from all symptoms. Her good health has lasted until now, more than seven years later.

Case 58. A similar condition affected a thirty-year-old woman, a hairdresser, who had been suffering for more than two years from painful attacks in the spine of her neck with radiation into the head and the right shoulder. The attacks were so violent that the patient had finally been forced to give up her job. All the treatments she had been receiving, including novocain injections, had not helped.

I found that the patient's menstruation had become more scanty during the last few years. Previously, it had lasted five days, now, only two. In connection with that, she had also put on weight. A reducing cure was prescribed and two artificial rashes, at intervals of one week, were applied. After that, the patient was free of complaints for four months. In this case, the treatment had to be repeated two to three times a year, whenever the pain reappeared. The menstruation was also corrected. Managing this way, the patient remained permanently able to work. She no longer had any serious attacks.

Arthritis of the spine of the chest (thorax)

Pain in the spine of the chest in younger people arouses the suspicion of tuberculosis of the bones. But in what medicine calls "common arthritis of the spine of the chest," there are no tuberculous complications.

In the common arthritis condition, patients complain of increasing stiffness, pain, and fatigue in the whole trunk. Lying down getting up, even rest in bed are accompanied by steady pain. Radiating neuralgic pain in chest and abdomen, in the arms and legs may develop and make even breathing difficult.

The usual treatment not only fails to improve or to cure such patients, but often also leads to the depressive prospect of permanent invalidism, an existence in a wheel chair.

In this area, too, proper counter-irritation and general care often bring such rapid improvement and cure that the whole picture is changed.

A few examples will serve as demonstration:

Case 59. A twenty-year-old mother had been suffering since the delivery of her second child from increasing pain, stiffness, and extreme fatigue of her whole spine. She could not bend down at all any longer. She was also unable to take her child up into her arms. Sitting down and getting up from a chair were agonizing. Even rest in bed was painful.

From the very beginning of her sickness, she had been treated with novocain injections, diathermy, hormones, vitamins, preparations of salicylates, and vaccines by the best available specialists, yet without any relief. Finally, she was told that the disease was irresistibly progressive, that she had even to resign herself to giving up the management of her own home and children. Considering her husband's modest salary and the impossibility for her of engaging hired help, her illness was indeed a family catastrophe.

Discouraged to the point almost of desperation, she came from Chicago to New York, recommended by a patient I had cured. My examination revealed, first of all, that her menstruation had become scanty since her last delivery. I found also a dilated, flabby stomach, and symptoms of extreme fatigue.

Intensive counter-irritation, combined with a regime for strengthening the stomach and general tonifying treatment resulted, within three weeks, in such an improvement that the patient was capable of resuming all her normal activities. She would have no difficulty in doing her housework or in caring for her children. She was so elated, I remember, she went dancing on her last evening before her return to Chicago.

The following case history is equally significant:

Case 60. A thirty-eight-year-old woman, doing the very strenuous work of superintendent in a large apartment house in addition to managing her own home, had been suffering for two and a half years from arthritis of the entire spine (the neck down to the sacral bone), with pains radiating into the arms and shoulders.

She had been treated in one of the best hospitals in New York, one with a special reputation for the cure of chronic diseases.

All possible diagnostic methods had been applied. The patient was also examined by experts in almost every clinical specialty, "in order to find the real cause of the disease."

Her tonsils were removed, physical therapy and various injections were prescribed. All these methods failed. Finally, she was put into the harnesslike corset of steel and leather, reaching from the shoulders down to the thighs. She was also told to give up her work and to take a complete rest.

The medical certificate from the hospital stated that she was "completely incapable of working" and that she would "never be able to support herself." The disease was diagnosed as "an irresistibly progressive and incurable condition."

My examination revealed, as in so many similar cases, too scanty menstruation during the last few years and moderate obesity. The X-ray examination showed an undoubted arthritis of the spine (spondylitis) of a medium degree.

Intensive counter-irritation combined with a mild reducing cure achieved within six weeks complete freedom from pain. The patient was able again not only to take care of her own household but also to return to her work as superintendent. The corset was dropped after the first week of treatment. She never wore it again. As of this date, nine years later, no relapse has occurred.

Three cases of arthritis of the spine that I treated during the last few years were particularly impressive. Each case was referred to me by the previous patient, after a successful cure. All three of them had been diagnosed as incurable by noted experts.

Case 61. Mr. V., a fifty-year-old owner of a dry-cleaning store, had been suffering for seven years from arthritis of the entire spine, the neck down to the coccyx bone. All movements, such as walking, sitting, lying down, getting up, and bending were extremely painful; in bed, the patient could not find a comfortable position.

He had consulted a large number of outstanding specialists and had been treated in the best of the special clinics. All treatments, including cortisone, had not helped. He was told that the cause of the disease was not known and that therefore no "specific remedy" was available.

The patient was a fairly short man, weighing two hundred twenty-five pounds. I prescribed a reducing cure immediately, then applied artificial rashes, step by step, along the whole spine. The pain diminished from day to day, so much so that after one week the patient was free from pain. Because of his high blood pressure and his fullness of blood (plethora), I also performed a moderate venesection. After a treatment of three weeks, he felt completely well, was able to perform all movements, and went back to his home in Jamestown, New York. He was instructed to continue his reducing cure.

Four months later, he wrote to tell me that his weight had gone down to one hundred ninety-six pounds, that he had "never felt so well" in his life, and that he was able to occupy himself again with the various sports that were his hobbies. His health has now been good for eight years.

A similar course can be seen in the following case, referred by Mr. V., from the same town:

Case 62. A forty-year-old woman went through a premature artificial menopause through radiation with radium for irregular hemorrhages. Afterward, she put on weight and developed some unpleasant metabolic disturbances. A few years ago, she had also had an operation for gallstones. Arthritis of the spine developed with violent backache and radiation of the neuralgic pain along the ribs (intercostal neuralgia). To alleviate the lower backache condition, an artificial surgical stiffening of both sacroiliac joints was performed. The arthritis, nevertheless, continued to progress to the upper part of the back.

This patient, too, had consulted several important specialists and clinics. The experts declared again that there was no cure for this disease.

At the end of February, 1949, she came to New York to my care. I prescribed a reducing cure and applied artificial rashes gradually over the whole spine.

Within one week, the pain had disappeared and did not come back. To prevent a relapse, the artificial rash was repeated twice, at intervals of one week. The patient was discharged after a treatment of three weeks with instructions to continue her reducing cure. Over the last 8 years, she has reported regularly that she has remained continuously free from distress.

How important it is to apply *individualized general treatment* in arthritis cases! The following history will once more illustrate this:

Case 63. A thirty-seven-year-old woman had been suffering for four years from arthritis of the spine. All movements and, again, even rest in bed were painful. Routine treatment had not been successful.

In the middle of October, 1949, she came from Jamestown to New York to consult me. This time, I found a very emaciated patient. She weighed only ninety-six pounds, having lost fourteen pounds during the last few years.

Her menstruation had become strikingly scanty during the last year. She suffered, too, from a dilated, hyperacid, flabby (splashing) stomach, which was also considerably dropped. In addition, she was smoking more than ½ pack of cigarettes a day which, as I have explained earlier, also frequently contributes to the origin of arthritis.

She was strictly advised to stop smoking. The tonifying diet for the stomach (previously described), together with tonic bitters, was prescribed. Once a week, an artificial rash over the whole spine was applied.

The condition of the patient improved rapidly. She gained nine pounds in three weeks. She was able to go home free from all pains. I receive reports from her regularly. She has been well now for more than seven years.

Arthritis of the lower (lumbar) spine, the sacral bone, and the coccyx bone

FREQUENT INVOLVEMENT OF THE SACROILIAC JOINT
AND THE SCIATIC NERVE

Arthritis of the lower spine occurs much more often than that of the upper part. Inflammatory changes with deposits in this region cause pain, stiffness, and restricted mobility. Here again, the usual routine treatment either fails completely or succeeds only after many months and years. The present erroneous concept about the cause of this condition—either an infection or a mechanical factor, such as a slipped disc—is, I believe, the reason for lack of success in treatment. It is the metabolic waste products that are the cause of the arthritis here, as in other locations. Treatment based on this concept has been much more successful.

A few case histories will illustrate this:

Case 64. A fifty-two-year-old construction worker had been suffering for five years from violent lower backache and sciatica. For two years, he was no longer able to work; his wife had to go to a factory to help support the family.

After numerous frustrating attempts with private physicians, he was admitted to a large chronic disease hospital in New York. All possible methods of examination were explored. Bony outgrowths or ruptured intervertebral discs, highly popular medical concepts at the time, were especially suspected. For this diagnosis, air inflations were made into the spinal canal and the patient nearly died of breath paralysis. The suspicions could not be verified, however, and the patient was finally told that the cause of his illness could not be sufficiently traced to help him.

My examination revealed moderate obesity, uric-acid diathesis, arthritis of the lumbar spine, and sciatica. Intensive counter-irritation of the skin and methods correcting the metabolism brought about a quick improvement. After a few weeks, the patient was able to resume his job as a construction worker. It is now more than ten years since I treated him. He is still climbing on roof-tops and lifting heavy beams without any difficulty. No relapse has occurred.

I have often found arthritic conditions of this type in middle-aged men who are heavy smokers.

Case 65. A fifty-six-year-old banker had been suffering for a year and a half from increasing lower backache with sciatica on his left side. The most outstanding specialists in New York had been consulted. Again, they were looking for possible ruptures of intervertebral discs which, if verified, would require an operation; in the meantime, the patient wore a heavy corset.

On taking over the treatment, I found a moderate obesity as well as uric-acid diathesis. To keep from gaining more weight, the patient had been smoking a great deal, thus increasing his disposition to arthritis and rheumatism. Other cases have demonstrated the same point. A hectic manner of living made the situation still worse.

I prescribed a reducing cure, combined with proper internal medication and counter-irritation of the skin. Within three weeks, the patient was entirely free from pain. He no longer wore the corset, was able to return to all his normal activities.

His usual way of life included, unfortunately, too much smoking, too much rushing, etc., and a slight relapse occurred six months later. But this was repaired within two weeks. Since then, nine years have passed and the patient has remained consistently well.

Such cases are not isolated instances nor are they limited to my experience only. They have been confirmed by many of my associates and followers for many years. When I was still practicing in Vienna, Dr. Karliner, an associate of mine now living in New York, told me the following remarkable story:

Case 66. A forty-five-year-old merchant came from Poland to Vienna to seek help for his lower backache, which had been persisting for two years with increasing pain. Bending down was totally impossible and other movements were very painful. The best specialists in Poland and Vienna could not provide him with any relief. The X-ray pictures had led to the diagnosis of "destructive arthritis" with beginning formation of stiffening bridges between the single vertebrae.

Dr. Karliner applied two artificial rashes with an interval of one week between them. A reducing cure for overweight was prescribed and a venesection, because of the fullness of blood, was performed. After the first artificial rash, the patient was able to bend down sufficiently to touch the floor with his finger tips. Within two weeks, he returned home completely cured.

The following case referred to me by the banker mentioned in Case 63 is also very characteristic.

Case 67. A forty-seven-year-old bank clerk who smoked two packs of cigarettes daily had been suffering from arthritis of the lower back for four years. During the night, when turning in bed, he often cried aloud from pain. He suffered severe attacks three to four times a year. During the attacks, he felt as if he were paralyzed, was confined each time to bed for several weeks, and was in danger of losing his job.

At the beginning of January, 1951, his employer suggested that he consult me. Chronic nicotine poisoning was evident; none of the former physicians he had seen had informed him of this. The patient could not cut out smoking completely but he was able to cut down considerably. Intensive counter-irritation of the skin on his back and both thighs was applied.

One week after the start of the treatment, he commented, "I think you've given me a new pair of legs." After two weeks, the patient was able to walk long distances and to perform the most strenuous gymnastic exercises. In order to prevent a relapse, I continued the treatment for two months.

I presented this patient two months later, together with similarly cured patients, at a medical meeting of the Stuyvesant Polyclinic in New York. The patient came by foot, purposely, from his office to the hospital, a distance of half an hour, to demonstrate his good physical condition. The patient has remained free from complaints ever since.

Case 68. A forty-three-year-old cutter in a clothing factory had been suffering for two years from pain in the lower spine. Previously, he had complained of arthritis of the shoulder. He, too, was a heavy smoker. For his backache, he wore a heavy corset. He was often unable to work.

Counter-irritation and saline laxatives improved the condition within four weeks so much that the patient was able to work steadily without complaints and without wearing a brace. Until now, for more than four years, the patient has been feeling fine.

Case 69. A thirty-five-year-old factory worker had been suffering for five years from arthritis of both sacroiliac joints, with pains radiating into the legs. Frequent attacks of paralyzing pain incapacitated him for work. Repeated treatment in hospitals did not bring any permanent relief. He, too, had to wear a heavy corset.

In May, 1951, he came under my care. I found moderate obesity and prescribed a reducing cure. Intensive counter-irritation of the skin was applied. After two weeks, the patient was able to drop the brace and to resume his work. After two months, he was discharged as cured. He has remained cured until now, more than five years later.

Lumbago (*Dragon's shoot*)

This very frequent form of lower backache concerns the soft parts (muscles and ligaments) more than the bones and joints. It is the kind of pain that often comes suddenly and has a paralyzing effect; it is therefore nicknamed Dragon's shoot. Draught, drenching, cold, or a sudden wrong movement is believed to be the causative factor. The usual treatment with heat, liniments, massage, and aspirin is lengthy and unreliable. Patients are often confined to bed for days, sometimes even for weeks; every movement may cause agonizing pain. Many explanations and treatments have been offered, most of them unsatisfactory.

On the other hand, one single well-applied artificial rash usually succeeds so quickly that some patients can get up the very next day and move around. A complete cure usually does not take longer than three to eight days. In order to prevent relapses, general factors such as overweight, fullness of blood, and uric-acid diathesis have to be taken care of.

I quote the following two examples:

Case 70. A forty-nine-year-old woman who had gone through a hysterectomy at the age of thirty-two had been suffering from increasing rheumatic and arthritic symptoms in the whole body.

Overweight, fullness of blood, high blood pressure, and a hard of hearing condition had also developed, symptoms seen in many such cases of premature artificial menopause.

Finally, she caught cold and became sick with a severe lumbago. All the usual methods of treatment did not help. She was in bed three months when I was called in to take over the treatment.

I performed a moderate bloodletting and applied an artificial rash over the whole painful area. I also prescribed a reducing cure combined with laxatives to improve the metabolism.

Three days later the patient was free from pain and was able to walk around without any difficulty. This was after a sickness of three months.

Case 71. A woman, thirty years old, had already had three violent attacks of lumbago within one year. These attacks usually lasted four to six weeks. This time, she had already been in bed for five weeks.

After application of an artificial rash, the patient was able on the third day to walk around and to resume her household work. After one week, she was completely free from any pain.

Characteristically, her menstruation had become more scanty during the last few years, a condition that we also treated, in order to avoid relapses.

We can see that even such a common, trivial disease as lumbago often has deeper causes in the metabolism and in other sectors of the system. Patent medicines and one-sided specialistic treatment, therefore, are not sufficient. Manifold, practically effective, and thorough medical knowledge is necessary in such cases, just as well as in the treatment of arthritis and allied conditions in general.

16 *Rheumatism of the nervous system (palsies, neuralgias, neuritis)*

As we know now that rheumatism and chronic arthritis (or chronic gout) are caused much more often by curable disturbances of the metabolism than by infection or incurable degeneration, we will not be surprised to hear that such irritant metabolic products may settle down not only in the joints and muscles, but also in the nervous system.

◆

Inflammation of the brain and spinal cord

Many cases of acute and chronic inflammation of the brain and of the spinal cord, whose cause is considered at present to be unknown (or rather forgotten) and which therefore are considered to be difficult to cure or incurable, were interpreted by our medical predecessors as gouty or rheumatic deposits and were also cured accordingly.

Even such serious conditions as Parkinson's disease (shaking palsy of the brain) and multiple sclerosis of the spinal cord, as well as similar ailments, occasionally may be considerably improved or arrested by methods of derivation and elimination, which improve the metabolism, as I have seen in my own experience. Much useful research work can be done in this direction.

In the peripheral nervous system neuritis (inflammation of the nerve) and neuralgias are very well-known diseases. The terms sciatica, neuritis of arms and legs, neuralgias of the face (trigeminus neuralgia, and neuralgias along the ribs (intercostal neuralgia) with and without preceding shingles (herpes zoster) are very familiar to all of us.

On the basis of the present conception one looks after infectious foci, and if one cannot find any bacteria as culprits, one takes refuge in recent years in the supposition of a still unknown virus (that is a fluid filterable infectious matter, which was previously called miasma). But all that blocks the way to a successful cure. The present usual treatment with vaccines, diathermy, short wave, X rays, and various injections is lengthy, uncertain, and frequently disappointing. Finally one consoles himself that nature herself may accomplish a cure. This, however, often means an agony lasting for months and years. For such an attitude one would not need any physicians at all.

If, however, one follows the advice of earlier physicians and the methods similar to the old procedures in a more modern form as they are described in this book, one may accomplish in most cases quick and lasting healing results. Most impressive for this purpose are counter-irritation of the skin and the methods of elimination that alter the metabolism in a favorable way. Patients who had been suffering for months and years from pain in their nerves usually can be freed from pain in a few days or weeks for good.

In previous chapters we have told how frequently such patients, after having been disappointed by scientific medicine, turned to lay healers and medical outsiders, by whom they were usually cured in a surprising way through the application of the old and forgotten methods of healing. We may mention on this occasion again the internationally known Dr. Munari in Treviso (Italy), Dr. Jetel in Vienna, Monsignor Kneipp in Germany, and many other less known healers in other countries.

We have made it our task for more than thirty years to re-introduce these very effective and therefore indispensable methods of healing and to make them a common good of all physicians and patients. However, even today a great effort is required to overcome the ultraconservative prejudice of official university medicine.

Sciatica

If someone has an acute or chronic attack of sciatica, the present-day official medical trend is, if possible, to find a mechanical or anatomic cause, e.g., pressure upon the nerve by bony outgrowths, slipped intervertebral discs, and the like. Tuberculosis of the bones and tumors are rare exceptions. We believe, however (again in agreement with earlier medical experience), that the everyday cases of sciatica are caused by arthritic or rheumatic metabolic disturbances. The disease therefore most often occurs in persons of middle or advanced age, who suffer from uric-acid diathesis and often enough at the same time complain of arthritis. In younger individuals, sciatica may be caused by occasional factors such as a drenching, catching a cold, draught, etc.

The present usual treatment consists of heating cabinets, diathermy, massage, aspirin, radiation, but is often lengthy, so that the painful condition may last many weeks, months, and even years.

We may recall the drastic example of the Swedish carpenter (case 64) who had been suffering from sciatica for five years, in spite of intensive specialistic treatment even in hospitals, and who had been cured within a few weeks permanently by our method.

As a home remedy one may try the compresses of benzine or kerosene along the whole course of the nerve, and one may also apply mustard plaster.

Most advantageous, certain, and quick is the application of an artificial rash over the whole painful area. In recent cases often a single application is sufficient. In chronic cases the procedure has to be repeated several times (about two to four times), at intervals of a week each time. In order to prevent a relapse and to accomplish a permanent cure, of course, the basic metabolic disturbance (e.g., overweight, uric-acid diathesis, fullness of blood, high blood pressure, chronic indigestion, constipation, diseases of the gallbladder, insufficient perspiration of the skin, or inadequate menstruation) must be carefully treated.

Besides the cases mentioned already, we may report, among a large number of successful cures, the following examples:

Case No. 72. A seventy-three-year-old business woman in Vienna had been suffering for seven weeks from a violent sciatica of the right leg, which forced her to stay home.

All the usual treatments, including injections of novocain into the nerve and even into the spinal cord, did not help. As she had to make an urgent business trip abroad, a quick cure was urgently required.

For these reasons we applied an artificial rash over the whole painful area and moreover prescribed an emetic, in order to accelerate the alteration of the metabolism. Within four days the patient was free from pain and was able to walk without any difficulty. In order to avoid a relapse, a reducing cure (as she was overweight) was prescribed, combined with saline laxatives, in order to improve her metabolism.

Case No. 73. The fifty-six-year-old wife of an important banker in Vienna had been putting on weight heavily since her menopause, and also complained of increasing rheumatic symptoms in the whole body. During the last few years also repeated attacks of sciatica with increasing violence occurred. The last attack had already lasted seven months.

The pain was so violent that the patient had to stay in bed during this whole period of time and she lamented loudly. In spite of the best treatment by specialists and visits to health resorts, no relief.

We applied an artificial rash and prescribed a reducing cure with intensive purgation by proper laxatives.

After two weeks the patient came to my office and presented herself as completely free from complaints. During the last four years, as long as I could follow up the patient, no relapse.

That sciatica is often only a partial symptom of a general gouty or uric acid diathesis may be seen by the following case.

Case No. 74. The secretary of a very high-ranking and even internationally known statesman in the old Austrian monarchy was a fifty-three-year-old woman whose black hair had turned white at the age of thirty-six, which always indicates nervous, glandular, or metabolic disturbances. She had been suffering for several years from chronic gout in her hands and feet, which were very painful. In connection with this condition, she had also several attacks of lumbago and sciatica, each lasting several weeks.

It is also very significant that the patient had to go repeatedly to Karlsbad on account of gallstone colics. Moreover, she had been suffering from overweight and too high blood pressure (180). The symptoms of the menopause appeared in the form of "terrible" flushes, after which she had been dripping wet from sweat, having also the sensation of palpitations in her heart.

All the usual treatments did not help.

A reducing cure, several bloodlettings (venesections), artificial rashes, and other procedures to improve the metabolism rendered the patient completely free from distress within two months.

Case No. 75. The thirty-six-year-old wife of an industrialist in Vienna had been suffering for four years from repeated attacks of sciatica. During her summer vacation in the vicinity of Salzburg she had been using the local natural baths, consisting of a strong solution of rock salt. Nevertheless she had such a violent attack of sciatica, not to be soothed by anything, that she returned to Vienna in great haste.

It had been overlooked that the patient had been suffering from a moderate obesity (overweight) but also from fullness of blood (plethora). A venesection (bloodletting), a reducing cure with purgative remedies and an artificial rash, removed the pain so quickly that the patient was able to return after one week of treatment to her summer resort and could attend the Salzburg festivals.

As patients who suffer from paralyzing sciatic pains may sometimes be so situated that a quick cure within a few days is required, the following case history may also be mentioned:

Case No. 76. A forty-eight-year-old woman was to travel within a week by airplane from New York to Paris. Unfortunately she had such a violent attack of sciatica that she was as though paralyzed, which of course made the possibility of the very important and urgent trip very questionable.

After having tried all the usual home remedies (sweating, aspirin, massage, liniments) and injections without results, the patient came under our care. In order to accomplish a quick cure, in this case we prescribed syrup of ipecacuanha as an emetic and applied an artificial rash over the whole painful area. After three days, the patient was able to walk around, and after one week she was completely free from complaints and was able to make the trip without any difficulty.

We may also remember the speedy cures achieved by the use of emetics reported earlier.

Neuralgia of the shoulder and arm

We have mentioned in the discussion of arthritis of the shoulder that there is not only always a circumscript disease of the mucous bursa (bursitis) or of the whole joint alone, but that the harmful metabolic products may also settle down on the surrounding muscles, ligaments, tendons, and nerves.

Three large cords of nerves pass by the shoulder joint, reaching down to the finger tips. The radialis nerve supplies, besides the upper arm and forearm, particularly the part of the hand situated near the thumb. The ulnaris nerve ends on the side of the little finger, and the medianus nerve has its final branches in the middle fingers.

Each single one, or all three of these nerves, may become inflamed and one calls that neuritis or neuralgia. Such pains are extremely agonizing and cause sleepless nights, in spite of the strongest sedatives.

The present generally used treatment all over the world is lengthy and usually ineffective, so that the ailment may last many weeks and months, sometimes even years.

Under the erroneous supposition that an infection may be the cause, this condition usually is treated with bacterial vaccines, however mostly without success.

In contrast to that this painful condition can usually be cured within one to three weeks by artificial rashes over the whole painful area. Of course at the same time internal medication combating the inflammation and the disturbed metabolism must be used as they accelerate the cure and protect the patient from relapses.

Case 77.   From my recent experience, I may also mention the following significant case. A fifty-six-year-old woman had been suffering for four months from neuritis of the upper arm with "terrible" pains. The family doctor and a noted nerve specialist prescribed physical therapy, pain-soothing remedies, and injections of vaccine, but without relief any time during the four months.

I applied counter-irritation. One single artificial rash over the whole painful area accomplished a cure within a week and the patient could work again. For the symptoms of uric-acid diathesis, adequate general treatment was prescribed in order to avoid a recurrence.

Many similar reports can be found in my scientific textbook on arthritis.

◆

Intercostal neuralgia

(Neuralgia of the nerves running along the ribs)

All nerves that leave the spinal cord may become inflamed either at the roots or farther down in their course. This pain is often so terrible that patients become drug addicts; some are tempted to suicide.

Here, too, the usual treatment is lengthy and uncertain, but counter-irritation and treatment of the deeper causes in the metabolism usually bring quick relief. The disease can almost always be cured in one to two weeks, sometimes even within three days.

Here are two case histories:

Case 78. A forty-eight-year-old woman had been having, during the last two years, repeated attacks of neuralgia along the ninth rib. The pain was so violent that none of the usual "pain killers" offered any relief. She was now taking morphine, her only solace. As happens often in diseases of this kind, I found that she also had other rheumatic and neuralgic symptoms in the rest of her body, particularly in her shoulders and knees. Repeated attacks of gallstone colic, obesity, and fullness of blood also clearly revealed a metabolic disturbance as the deeper cause of her neuralgia.

The usual treatment with heat, aspirin, injections, etc., did not help for it did nothing to improve her general condition.

I prescribed a reducing cure, moderate bloodlettings, and counter-irritation. The general condition improved quickly. The neuralgia disappeared permanently after a treatment of two and a half weeks.

Case 79. A forty-two-year-old woman had been suffering for three years from rheumatic pains in her arms and legs. During the last few months an intercostal neuralgia, corresponding to the sixth and seventh ribs on the left side, had also developed. The pain was violent and defied all the usual treatments.

It had again been overlooked that the patient was very much

overweight. This was apparently caused by too scanty menstruation; periods lasted only one day. Moreover, fullness of blood and uric-acid diathesis were evident.

A reducing cure, bloodletting, and artificial rashes improved the condition considerably. But in this case it took five weeks longer before the patient was completely free from complaints. The usual healing time, according to my method, is one to two weeks only. The very deep-seated metabolic disturbance made more extensive treatment necessary here.

Herpes zoster (*shingles*)

Closely related to the intercostal neuralgia is the herpes zoster disease, more often referred to by the layman as "shingles." It consists of a very painful eruption of the skin in the form of small vesicles along one or several intercostal nerves.

Present-day medicine attributes the cause to a still unknown virus. The idea of a disturbed metabolism is equally possible and much easier to handle. Actually, the treatment based on the unknown virus theory, by injections and radiation, is unreliable, permitting this very painful condition to last many weeks and even many months.

My method, by applying anti-inflammatory remedies, such as mild preparations of mercury and antimony, supplemented by bloodletting and blistering, shortens the duration of the treatment to one or two weeks.

If the condition is left to the self-healing power of nature alone (the expectative treatment), the vesicular rash dries up after a few weeks. But then it frequently leaves behind a most painful neuralgia that may last many months and even years. I saw such a patient only recently:

Case 80.   A sixty-five-year-old man had suffered a most severe attack of shingles on the left side of his chest six months before. The pain was so violent that his physician considered the possibility of a stomach ulcer. The patient himself was afraid he had heart disease.

Treatment with dusting powder, injections, short waves, and X rays dried the rash up within a few weeks. But it left behind brown spots on the skin and a violent neuralgia, which defied all treatment.

Although the physician had taken into account the possibility of a stomach ulcer and hyperacidity of the stomach was found to exist, nothing constructive was done about this. Routine treatment with milk, bland diet, etc., was of no help. The patient's uric-acid diatheses was not considered.

My prescription of a tonic diet and stomach bitters, combined with proper alkalizers and, most important, the application of an artificial rash (this time in imitation of nature, which had produced blisters in the form of shingles), removed the neuralgia permanently within two weeks.

Many similar cases are reported in my scientific textbook on arthritis.

Neuralgia of the face (trigeminal neuralgia)

Neuralgia of the face has always been known as one of the most violent and unbearable forms of pain. Since it originates in any of the three branches of the fifth nerve coming from the brain (nervus trigeminus), the forehead and the eye, the cheeks and the nose, or the mouth and the chin may be involved.

Drugs, radiations, and injections have proved disappointing in most cases. The disease may last for many months and years. In order to stop the severe pain, physicians have tried to block the various branches of the nerves by anesthesia or to destroy them by chemical means (e.g., with the injection of alcohol) or by surgery, where the painful branches of the nerve are actually severed. Some surgeons have even resorted to removing the common root (ganglion) of all the three branches on the base of the brain, a very serious and dangerous major operation.

In all these surgical procedures, the unpleasant consequence of paralysis of the muscles of one side of the face and loss of sensation occurs, especially disturbing in the region of the eye, where it leads to dryness, inflammation, and ulceration of the surface of the eyeball.

Fortunately, an understanding of the deep-seated, general disturbances, such as chronic gout, uric-acid diathesis, etc., as the causative factors in this illness, makes a real cure possible. I have achieved relatively quick cures with proper internal medication and correct external applications. The quick pain-soothing effect of vesication, by plaster of Spanish fly or by artificial rashes on the painful spot, has been particularly amazing.

I would like to cite two such typical cases from my own experiences:

Case 81. A forty-five-year-old woman had been suffering for four years from violent attacks of trigeminal neuralgia, which occurred most often at the time of her menstruation. The neuralgia corresponded to the second and third branch of the nerve on the right side (involving the upper and lower jaw).

Because of the jaw involvement, she had, upon medical advice, had four of her teeth extracted. It did not give her any relief. All the other usual treatments had also failed. Now an operation was being planned.

Her case history revealed the interesting fact that she had had, four and a half years ago, a stubborn rash on her face, which healed up after a treatment of several months. Apparently, it had left behind a violent neuralgia. This was, I thought, a significant factor. And I proceeded accordingly.

I applied an artificial rash over the whole painful area and put a blistering plaster of Spanish fly behind the right ear. I also prescribed certain laxatives to cleanse the system of irritant metabolic waste products. To my own surprise, the pain disappeared permanently within a week. This result is logical, however, as counterirritation also cures all other forms of neuralgia.

The connection of trigeminal neuralgia with arthritis, uric-acid diathesis, and other general disturbances can be seen in the following case history:

Case 82. A forty-six-year-old stout, dark-haired woman had been suffering from repeated attacks of gallstone colic, flabbiness of the stomach, itching over the whole body, mental depression, and rheumatic pain in her thumb. Later on, a cramplike pain in the right cheek (tic convulsif), corresponding to the second branch of the facial nerve, also developed.

Radiation with X rays and diathermy applied for several weeks did not help. The pain was so excruciating that the patient wanted to kill herself. Suicidal attempts occur often in patients suffering from trigeminal neuralgia.

I applied an artificial rash over the whole painful area and prescribed an emetic or vomiting drug. I added sweating procedures and other measures to improve the metabolism. After one week, the patient was free from pain.

Neuralgia of the head

Neuralgia, particularly in the back of the skull (occiput), but also in other parts of the head, may also occur. The causes of these neuralgias are similar to those in other nerve pains. They, too, can be quickly cured by the same methods, particularly through counter-irritation of the skin.

Polyneuritis (general inflammation of the nerves)

Pain, numbness, paralysis, and weakness in the nerves of the arms, the legs and the trunk may all appear at the same time. This condition is called polyneuritis. Since common remedies and physical therapy usually fail, such patients feel steadily sick and are often chronic invalids. How ironically inadequate the usual treatment can be may be learned from a consultation that I had more than twenty-five years ago in Vienna with one of the most famous professors of internal medicine in Europe. The fifty-one-year-old patient had gone through a hysterectomy at the age of forty-six and had been suffering from a painful polyneuritis, particularly in her arms and legs. After a thorough examination, the professor prescribed salol, which is close to aspirin. Of course, this did not help at all for it was not treating the uric-acid diathesis, so often a condition in the menopause.

Energetic attempts to improve and to clean the metabolism by sweating cabinets, saline laxatives, and mild preparations of mercury and antimony finally cured the condition.

Almost always, certain general disturbances can be found in such cases of polyneuritis, e.g., overweight, fullness of blood, insufficient perspiration of the skin, too scanty menstruation in younger women, disturbances of the menopause, uric-acid diathesis, and chronic gout. Exaggerated smoking and alcoholism are also frequent causative factors. Infection is very rarely a cause. Only if the individual's general condition is properly taken care of can one expect a cure. Wonder drugs or patent medicines are useless.

Inflammation of the tendon sheets, bursae, and
muscles, including muscle cramps

The tendency to find, wherever possible, a local anatomic change, with an appropriate name, has led to the idea of considering the inflammation of certain mucous sacs (bursae) as a special disease, now called "bursitis" and separated from the arthritic condition to which it usually belongs. If calcium deposits are found in the X-ray picture of such a bursitis, many physicians believe that these calcifications or even the whole sac must be surgically removed. But, usually, the rest of the joint with its surroundings is also sick and a much more thorough treatment is necessary. I have quoted such a case (No. 35). Counter-irritation and proper general care usually cure this condition in a short time and make an operation unnecessary. The same holds true for bursitis on the knee, the elbow, the heel, etc.

Inflammation of the tendon sheets on the forearm and fingers

This condition occurs particularly often in piano- and violin-players through overexertion. In later stages of life, tendovaginitis may also be caused by uric-acid diathesis.

With the common general treatment, such a disease may last several months and even years, thus incapacitating the patient, who had to cancel whole concert seasons.

On the other hand, artificial rashes and blistering plasters on the painful spot, combined with proper general care, have made possible the cure of many such patients in a few weeks. A number of these cures are described in my scientific textbook on arthritis.

Muscular rheumatisms (sometimes also inflammations of the muscles, myositis)

These are usually collectively called rheumatism of the muscles. They may appear in an acute or chronic form and may last a long time if energetic local treatment (particularly counter-irritation) and treatment for general improvement of the metabolism are not undertaken.

Sweating procedures and bloodletting in its various forms are often necessary to accelerate the healing. I have quoted in other writings many similar cures.

Muscular cramps

This is also considered a difficult problem in modern medicine and may truly be so if we do not look for the causes in the metabolism of the body. Most frequently, they occur as cramps of the muscles of the neck. This condition can become most annoying in its persistent form of a wry neck, that is a twisted fixation of the neck and head in a wrong position owing to a lasting contraction of the muscles. Fortunately the "wry neck" condition is rare for it is indeed difficult to cure! Physicians sometimes resort to surgery by severing the spastic muscles. There are, however, several other means that can be tried before surgical interference is carried out, for example vomiting as a kind of shock treatment. Bloodletting or artificial rashes *may* loosen the spastic condition.

I observed a patient who had been suffering from such a wry neck condition for a year and a half. Nobody could help him. Even the methods I suggested and tried did not bring relief. The patient finally went to a particularly skilled chiropractor who cured him permanently within three weeks. Chiropractors generally promise more than they can do, particularly in the field of arthritis. But in this particular case, there can be no doubt that chiropractic manipulation was the only thing that helped.

Another characteristic form of muscular cramps is the cramp in the calves. These spasms either attack the patients at night with violent pain or force them, when walking on the street, to stop short suddenly. Patients then begin to limp. This condition is called "intermittent claudication."

Many explanations have been given for this striking symptom. It usually concerns middle-aged or elderly people, particularly men who are heavy smokers. Hardening of the arteries is considered by some as the cause, an irreparable one. As such, the condition has been called "Buerger's disease." On the supposition that the nerves are causing the cramps, the French surgeon, Leriche, tried performing operations consisting of peeling the arteries completely out of their surrounding tissues. The purpose was to sever, in this way, the supplying nerves. Such a drastic operation can be avoided.

Earlier medical systems and my own practical experience seem to indicate, however, that the cramps do not come from the wall of the blood vessels but from their contents, the blood, which is overcharged with irritant waste products. Consequently, in most cases such operations can be avoided, sometimes even by a simple bloodletting (venesection) or by artificial rashes over the involved area. There is also an analogy in the condition to other forms of cramps in the blood vessels and muscles owing to irritant metabolic waste products, e.g., spasms of the coronary arteries of the heart (angina pectoris). These can be eliminated easily and with lasting effect in the ways I have described in my textbook.

Middle-aged and elderly people often complain of numbness and other abnormal sensations in their fingers, toes, arms, and legs, and sometimes even of very painful cramps of the blood vessels (vascular spasms). Here, again, the present trend of scientific medicine makes hardening of the arteries and irritation of the pertaining nerves responsible for these cramps, again a most pessimistic outlook. Earlier medical systems, based on the principle of the pathology of the fluids, looked for the cause here, too, not in the walls of the arteries, but in their contents, the blood. By cleaning the blood of those irritant metabolic products that provoke the cramps, all these abnormal and annoying sensations can be removed. Sweating, purging, carefully planned bloodletting, and a large number of "blood-purifying" remedies have proved effective in most cases.

17 *Gout and rheumatism in other organs*

The same metabolic disturbances that we have observed in the joints, the nerves, the muscles, and other parts of the organs of the locomotion system may also involve the inner organs, such as heart, lungs, pleura, liver, and kidneys, and the organs of sense. Earlier physicians frankly spoke of gouty or rheumatic deposits in these inner organs; modern medicine looks rather for infectious or anatomical degenerative causes. The conception of the earlier physicians simplifies the treatment, however, and more important, yields better practical results.

Gouty and rheumatic diseases of the organs of sense

All five organs of sense may be damaged by gouty, arthritic, and rheumatic morbid substances.

The sense of touch can be affected in cases both of polyneuritis and of inflammations of single nerves.

The senses of smell and taste may become lost, particularly often after artificially induced, premature menopause, a condition in which rheumatism, inflammation of the joints, and of the nerves may spread over the entire body. Improvement of the metabolism here, too, often helps to accomplish a cure where overspecialized medicine remains ineffective.

Diseases of the eye

Modern ophthalmology has made great headway in the diagnosis and surgical treatment of eye diseases. But it has not yet sufficiently progressed either in effectively preventing many inflammatory, degenerative eye processes or in finding a conservative cure for them.

Glaucoma (the green cataract), for example, was considered by earlier medicine as a "gout attack" of the eye, and therefore often successfully treated with local and general bloodlettings, counter-irritation of the surrounding skin, and many anti-inflammatory internal remedies that improved the overcharged metabolism at the same time. The same procedures can still, particularly if treatment starts in the earlier stages of the disease, often avoid mutilating operations (cutting out a section of the iris). Characteristically, patients suffering from glaucoma complain of high blood pressure, arthritis, and other related conditions which, all together, point to harmful metabolic waste products, most of which can be eliminated. (I have had favorable experiences of my own, under control of eye specialists.)

Similar considerations are valid also for the common cataract (gray cataract). Persons with uric-acid diathesis and those who have wasted their vital forces early in life have a particular disposition for early and severe cataracts.

In most cases, cataract occurs in the advanced years of life, that is in the sixth, seventh, or eighth decade. The progress of the disease, however, can often be arrested by a regime that cleans the metabolism.

I have seen a number of patients in whom reliable eye specialists found a beginning or moderately progressed cataract. These patients were told that they would need an operation in one or two years. A regime to improve the metabolism has very often succeeded in keeping the opacity (dimness) of the lenses from progressing, and an operation was avoided.

But when the opacity of the lenses is too far advanced, an operation (removal of the opaque lens) should be performed. With refined modern techniques, it gives splendid results.

Numerous other diseases of the eye—for example, acute and chronic "rheumatic" inflammation of the iris (iritis) or of the sklera (skleritis), and of the cornea as well as that of deeper layers of the eyeball—are not necessarily caused by infection, as is still widely believed. They can be provoked by irritant rheumatic or gouty metabolic products as we so frequently find them in middle-aged or elderly persons. The same holds true for the inflammation of the retina (retinitis), the optic nerve, and the chorea (chorioiditis). Against all these conditions, modern medicine is rather helpless for it does not see the causative factors. General anti-inflammatory methods, however, which at the same time clean the metabolism of irritant waste products, may improve or cure these conditions.

Detachment of the retina (ablatio retinae), which often leads to blindness and is principally due to high blood pressure and fullness of blood, can frequently be prevented by taking care of the general cause in the circulatory system. Bloodletting (local and general) and similar methods are helpful and should be attempted more often by modern eye specialists as effective prevention and eventual cure. In advance cases Gonin's operation gives splendid results.

Diseases of the ear

Like eye diseases, the diseases of the ear are also frequent in middle-aged and elderly people. I am not including, of course, the acute inflammatory and the scrofulous or tuberculous ear diseases of childhood and adolescence.

The reason is again the accumulation of irritant metabolic products (such as uric acid, calcium salts, etc.) in the aging organism. Hard of hearing conditions, deafness, ringing and buzzing in the ear, as well as dizziness, are most often found in persons after the age of fifty. Modern specialization frequently attributes these to irreparable anatomic damage. Earlier medicine preached and modern constitutional therapy successfully practices in such cases on the basis of improving the general metabolism and the local congestion.

Dizziness and noises in the ear, for example, can often be improved or cured by local or general bloodletting, also by counter-irritation behind the ears. Proper laxatives, sweating procedures, and last but not least, long-continued sneezing (through the use of snuff and the like) are often helpful. Similar views hold true for slight and medium hard of hearing cases. I have had many good results with such methods in my own practice, particularly with women after the change of life.

Rheumatic and gouty diseases of the inner organs

The anatomic and bacteriologic trend of the last hundred years has led to much too great a pessimism in the judgment and treatment of many internal diseases. Thus one speaks, for example of irreparable calcification or hardening of the arteries (arteriosclerosis) with high blood pressure. Modern constitutional therapy, agreeing with earlier medicine, considers irritant metabolic waste products (which can be removed) as a frequent *cause* of vascular cramps, embolisms, hemorrhages (e.g., into the brain), etc. Many "blood-purifying" drugs, proper diet, as well as carefully planned local and general bloodlettings (venesection, cupping, leeches), are at our disposal, and have enabled the followers of this trend to accomplish many unexpected healing results.

Cerebral stroke (hemorrhage into the brain) has increased in frequency during our century to an alarming extent—simply for the reason that the prevention and curative methods of general care, particularly bloodletting, have been neglected. Good physicians should notice the danger of stroke months and years in advance. They are then capable of preventing many premature deaths.

Even more startling are the frequent sudden deaths from heart attack, mostly because of angina pectoris and coronary thrombosis. More than a hundred years ago Hufeland, one of the most famous physicians of his time, was complaining that the medical decline of bloodletting was causing a surprising increase in deaths from heart attack and cerebral stroke. How much more reason he would have to be alarmed by the attitude of present-day medicine in this respect and by the results of this attitude!

If somebody complains today of angina pectoris, nitroglycerine and sedatives are usually prescribed. But nothing is done for the improvement of the quantity, quality, and distribution of blood, except for the prescription of digitalis and similar drugs.

Cleaning from the blood the irritant metabolic products that cause the vascular cramps and the embolisms is a method that cannot be ignored. A large variety of medicines useful for this purpose are available, particularly saltpeter, one of the seven arcana (fundamental remedies) of the earlier physicians.

Many diseases of the lung and the pleura (pleurisy) in which a bacteriological cause cannot be found with certainty may also be considered a consequence of gouty and rheumatic deposits and successfully treated by elimination and derivation.

Modern methods of killing the bacteria with sulfa drugs, penicillin, and other antibiotics have been highly successful in the treatment of pneumonia and pleurisy. The antibiotics may, however, leave behind unpleasant and often chronic aftereffects in cases where the metabolic products are the cause of the disease and have not been removed.

For many centuries, long before the antibiotics were discovered sweating and vesication with plasters of Spanish fly combined with internal anti-inflammatory remedies, such as saltpeter and ammonium chloride, were used very successfully. The best proce dure would, therefore, seem to be to combine these methods with the modern antibiotics.

Bronchial asthma may also often be caused by rheumatic or gouty deposits. The modern concept of infectious or allergic causes very frequently fails to provide good results. Improvement of the general metabolism is often more successful, particularly when an emetic is prescribed.

Finally, gallstones and kidneystones also belong to the group of gouty and arthritic diseases. The formation of stones in the gallbladder and kidney may occur in a way similar to the calcification that takes place in and around the joints. French medicine includes gallstones and kidneystones in the conception of "arthri-isme."

Actually, we find arthritis, high blood pressure, uric-acid diathesis, gallstones, and kidneystones combined strikingly often in the same person.

Many major operations on kidneys and gallbladder may be avoided if we improve the metabolism of the patient as a whole. It has been proved by reliable earlier observations and is being demonstrated today in certain health resorts that gallstones and kidneystones can be broken up into sand and eliminated through the bowels and the bladder. Quite a number of such resolving drugs are known to those who are familiar with earlier medicine.

final word

In contrast to the present widespread opinion that arthritis is difficult to cure or even incurable, I am in a position to prove that arthritis, rheumatism, and allied conditions such as neuralgias yield the most gratifying cures if we combine the modern analytic and theoretical approach with the practical and empirical methods of the past.

I have demonstrated that patients who had been treated for many months and even years without success by competent hospitals and specialists were freed from complaints by me in a few weeks, sometimes even in a few days. The methods I have used are fully and exactly described in this book.

Labeling a method "new" or "old" is not in any real sense of any consequence. What is important is what the method accomplishes. As one of our outstanding masters once said, "Healing and helping are the noblest parts of medicine."

PART THREE

HISTORICAL SURVEY

18 *The history of medicine as an indispensable source of knowledge to the practicing physician*

Whereas, up to a hundred years ago scientific medical education was based on the complete knowledge of practical historical facts, combined with the steady progress of medicine, today the methods of earlier physicians before our "truly scientific" era of experimental medicine are considered outmoded and useless. Often enough, they are even called superstitious, unscientific, and harmful, and therefore not worthwhile knowing and studying. But, as we have pointed out for many years, in numerous articles and several textbooks, this is a *grave error,* detrimental to our healing capacity.

Medical systems and methods, like styles and fashions, change through the ages. Each of these systems developed theories in order to interpret the processes of diseases and their cures, as well as *practical methods* that were *effective.* With the shift of theories, for instance, from humoral to cellular pathology, during the last hundred years, healing methods of earlier systems have been *discarded* almost completely although they were and are still more effective in certain diseases than our modern methods, based on experimental medicine. This applies to almost all branches of medicine. In fact, by radically discarding all so-called "empirical" methods of the past, which in reality are scientific methods according to earlier systems, we have *lost* nine out of ten parts of all available *healing power*.

These words are written with the hope of demonstrating this *alarming* fact by the example of arthritis and allied conditions. A brief historical survey will show how much we can *learn from* the writings of our medical *predecessors,* who, not only in the field of arthritis, but also in other realms of medicine often score surprising and quick results where the most sophisticated modern and scientific treatment fails.

The utilitaristic approach to the history of medicine must be a fundament of modern medical education, if, according to the words of Cushing, we would not arrive "at a blind alley." The unbiased "study of literature and of nature," as the great masters of the past put it, must again become the two main sources of our knowledge.

Prehistoric, primitive, and exotic medicine in the treatment of arthritis

There is a widespread belief that prehistoric, primitive, exotic, and folk medicine were mainly guided by superstition and magic and that therefore their procedures are no longer of any practical concern. But ethnologists, among them recently E. Ackerknecht, have stressed that besides the magicians, there was always another kind of "lower grade" medicine men, who applied practical and empirical methods of healing. It is those methods which in many instances remained unchanged until our day and still form a valid basis of all practical medicine.

It is common to those early and primitive trends of medicine that most diseases are considered to be something foreign to the body, demons as well as poison and corrupted body humors or other harmful substances. *Derivation* and *elimination* by all natural channels and other possible ways was the *keynote*. This should be, but no longer is, the basic motive of all sound practical medicine.

In the treatment of arthritis or rheumatism and allied conditions common to all primitive nations of the earth, we find the fundamental methods of purging, vomiting, sweating, bleeding, particularly cupping with scarification on the sick spot, and especially counter-irritation in all its forms (such as provoking redness, hyperemia, local hemorrhages in the skin, blisters, artificial rashes, and cauterization with hot fluids and solids, with chemical caustics, and finally with the hot iron) to be the most effective remedy.

◆

American Indians and their treatment of arthritis

According to Eric Stone's monograph: "Medicine Among The American Indians," edited by E. B. Krumbhaar (*Clio Medica*), 1932, Paul B. Hoeber, New York, the Red Indians of Northern America, in spite of their otherwise proverbial good health, suffered relatively often from rheumatism and arthritis on account of the rather rough and changing climate of this continent and because of their exposure to all kinds of weather, in hunting and warfare.

Stone claims that the Indians were keen observers and were adequate practitioners, so far as an empiric knowledge of disease would permit. They usually got along by treating the patients with drugs and physical therapy, in the majority of cases. "It was only when diseases failed to respond to these measures . . . that they had recourse to their more complicated magic rituals."

Among others they had a very effective *antirheumatic medicine*, consisting of six herbs.

For any form of gastric disorders they employed *emetics* as frequently as the white man takes laxatives. The medical lore was very rich in the emetic roots and herbs.

Stone writes: "Because of their diet and their constant exposure to the inclemencies of the weather, the American Indians were unusually prone to arthritis, rheumatism and neuritis. They considered the conditions as phases of a single disorder and used the identical treatment for all. Because of their prevalence, the Indians developed a considerable armamentarium for the relief of arthritis and allied conditions."

Internally they used jalap, cimicifuga, fuzzy weed (artemisia dracunculoides) and lead plant (amorpha canescens).

Externally they used balm of Gilead (pecca grandis), the bark of walnut, and wet dressings of petroleum.

I can confirm especially that jalap internally is very effective as an alterative laxative with systemic side effects in arthritis. Wet dressings with petroleum or its derivate, benzine, were still used by the European armies in the first World War as a very effective emergency treatment for lumbago, sciatica, neuritis, neuralgia, arthritis, and muscular rheumatism. I am still using it today in certain cases with surprising effects.

Other counter-irritants were freely used by the Red Indian such as the usual moxas as well as scarification combined with cupping. The crushed leaves of pulsatilla and other ranunculus species were applied to the skin over involved joints, and afforded a sufficiently strong counter-irritant to produce a large blister.

Fumigation of sick joints with the flowers of false lupine rapidly reduced the swelling and eased the pain. Also many kinds of washes and poultices were used.

Their moxa treatment of neuralgia was very effective.

It has been confirmed by many sources that tumors, particularly cancer, were almost unheard of.

Stone concludes that the Indians added fifty-nine drugs to our modern pharmacopeia, including cascara, condurango, and lobelia. "Their treatment of many conditions was equal to or better than that of the white physicians of the eighteenth century (e.g., wounds, fractures, and empyema)." We may add that *their trea-*

ment of arthritis, rheumatism and allied conditions was *more effective* in some respects *than ours is today.*

Medicine of the Far East

(Chinese, Japanese, Malayan, Tibetan, etc.)

According to historical sources Chinese scientific medicine and literature reaches back as far as 3000 or even 4000 B.C. If we abstain from magic, religious, and superstitious ingredients, the Chinese records tell us of many *successful cures* performed by internal and external treatment. *Internally* they usually applied herbs with definite alterative, purgative, diuretic, and sudorific effect. *Externally* two methods, apparently their own specific invention, are known, namely acupuncture and moxibustion, which later on were adopted by the Japanese and other neighboring nations.

These two methods have been proved very effective also in arthritis and rheumatism, as a kind of strong counter-irritation and reflexotherapy.

Moxibustion is a kind of cauterization with lighted (burning) flaxlike plant fibers, usually taken from certain species of the herb artemisia. From these dried plant fibers small cones are formed, drenched with a solution of saltpeter, put on the proper spot of the skin and lighted. They leave behind a small burn of the size of a pea, and according to modern medical travelers in the Far East, are amazingly beneficial even in severe cases of trigeminal neuralgia, sciatica, neuritis, arthritis, rheumatism, or allied conditions.

The location of these burns, usually several at a time, was chosen carefully according to long established laws of experience in a similar way as the fire surgery or "point de feu" of the Arabs and Hindus. These locations often corresponded to the zones of referred pain or Head's zones. But whereas today we use these reflectoric relations mostly for diagnostic purposes, the ancient nations used them in a centripetal way for effective *reflexotherapy*.

Still more mysterious is *acupuncture*. The Chinese had a large and intricate system of pricking the skin and deeper lying organs with fine needles of different sizes and shapes and made of different metals. The underlying anatomical and physiological reasoning was still more complicated and followed their specific ideas on vascular reflexes and vital currents in the nerves. Strange as this may sound, there is no doubt that they had *surprising results* in otherwise refractory cases, such as angina pectoris, asthma, palsies, pylorospasmus of the newborn, severe neuralgia, arthritis, and ankylosis. There are many European physicians who have been eyewitnesses to those results, among them a former student of mine, Dr. Miorini, formerly of Vienna, now for many years in Shanghai.

The Hospital Bellan, in Paris, had investigated and confirmed these methods for a number of years. It is said also that Yale University in this country has become interested in reinvestigation of these methods.

The *Malayans* in the Dutch East Indies, as I know also from reliable eyewitnesses, have a large catalogue of herbs, used externally as effective counter-irritants, provoking blisters and rashe and acting internally by their alterative, antidyscrasic, and especially antiarthritic effect. All these methods and means deserve a closer study.

African tribes

African Negroes in the bush use the leaves of certain species of aloes as an effective *counter-irritant* in arthritis, neuralgia, and rheumatism. But only the fresh sap of the plant is effective, if it is rubbed in, just as is poison ivy or rhus toxicodendron. The dried plant loses its effect.

Other tribes have developed a method *to cure neuralgia* by tattooing the painful area with certain thorns that discharge an irritant dyestuff.

◆

Hindu medicine

Our knowledge of ancient Hindu medicine is based for the most part on the writings of Susruta and Charaka, who lived about A.D. 500. I have used a Latin translation of the writings of Susruta (*Ayurvedas,* edited by Dr. F. Hessler, Erlangen, 1844). Hessler believed, and we think he is right, that the knowledge displayed in these writings goes back as far as at least a thousand years before Christ and that the Hindu doctrines are superior in some respects even to those of Hippocrates. In fact, if we study the three volumes of this quoted book, we find such an enormous refinement and so many analogies to Hippocratic ideas and sentences that it becomes doubtful whether Hippocrates did not learn many of his conceptions from oriental medicine, and especially from India.

It is exciting to read that they diagnosed diabetes mellitus and cured it definitely with bitumen (a fossil pitch found in the mountains). Their refined indications for purging, vomiting, venesection, leeches, cupping, cauterization, and numerous internal remedies are admirable.

Concerning *arthritis* and allied conditions they had also a well developed diagnosis and therapy. As in other ancient systems they believed that arthritis and rheumatism may originate from *a surplus* of bile, phlegm, blood, fat, or air. They distinguished between a superficial and a deep variety of the disease. The former manifested itself on the skin and the muscles, the latter on the nerves and joints. A large number of vegetable drugs to *clean from the system* these superfluous and harmful substances is quoted. As a main remedy the tasty resin Bdellium (resin of the wine palm) is praised, just as in earlier European medicine other resolvent, alterative, and purgative resins such as jalap and guajac have been used successfully. They knew the connection between arthritis and *renal calculi* and in contrast to present-day medicine, believed that they can be broken down to sand and thus eliminated, which is true and has been proved by many earlier physicians. They used for this purpose the seeds of Ruellia longifolia.

Furthermore, as a cure of arthritis they used systematic and individualized purgations, emetics, sweating, fumigation, liniments, and bleeding, especially leeches, venesections, cupping with scarification, and *cauterization*. The latter was used in different forms, among which are such chemicals as hot lye, prepared from the ash of certain plants; by hot oil; by glowing roots or, the strongest method, by hot iron. Fire as the "supreme remedy" was known to them as it was to Hippocrates. They believed "that there is only one still more powerful remedy, namely prayer." As preliminary steps of therapy they also quoted diet, drugs, and surgery.

For *internal treatment* of arthritis and allied conditions they used the root of Convolvulus Turpethum as one of the most effective purgatives. To *resolve the deposits* in the joints, and also renal calculi, they used a diluted solution of caustic lye, taken from the ash of certain plants, given internally as a potion over a longer period. Later physicians applied in a similar way solutions of different alkalies by mouth, which we find also in certain natural mineral waters.

The powerful "cleansing" effect of *emetics* was well known to the Hindus. Most commonly they used a decoction of the plant Vangueria spinosa. "After thorough vomiting, head and heart feel relieved and purged. The soul has a sense of well-being and serenity," reads one of their most famous sentences, a truth that deserves to be remembered again by modern medicine. In fact, vomiting is one of the most effective forms of natural shock treatment in early stages of mental diseases (see the author's *Textbook on Constitutional-Therapy*).

Concerning cauterization it reads: "Lixivio caustico gravior ignis in operationibus demonstratus est propterea, quod morbi igne adusti non rursus apparent et quod morbos medicamentis, scalpellis et lixivio caustico insanabiles sanat" (Susruta, *Liber Principiorum*, or *Sustrast hana*, Ch. 12, De ignis usu). In English: "Fire is more powerful than caustic lye because diseases treated with fire do not reappear. Fire cures such diseases as cannot be cured by drugs, by knife, and by caustic lye."

Among diseases that should be treated with *cauterization* Susruta quotes diseases of the head, the eyes, the skin, the rectum (hemorrhoids) and *joint diseases,* especially those forming nodes and deposits.

There is a special chapter on *arthritic nodes* in the second book of Susruta called *Sarirast' hana* (which means Somatology), Ch. 18 which reads: "Nodis arthriticis crudis médicus, praeceptorum gnarus, adhibeat curandi rationem in curandis intumescentiis adhibitam; et servet etiam semper hominis vim; quae servata vim morborum demit." In English: "In case of crude arthritic nodes the expert physician should apply the same methods as in curing tumors [swellings] in general; he should be careful to preserve the strength of the patient; in doing so he will diminish the disease." In other words, arthritic deposits have to be treated like other swellings, that is by adequate *general* and *local therapy.* General therapy consists in strengthening the whole body and in correcting faulty or superfluous humors by the different methods of alteration, resolution, and elimination. Locally sudorific ointments, as in the writings of Hippocrates leeches, cupping, and finally cauterization are recommended.

"Ustio enim saluti est." Translated: "Cauterization is beneficial."

Sweating also is advocated "Illinendo Curcumam anthorhizon, aut lacca usta sudor aegroti eliciendus est." Translated: "The physician should provoke sweat in the patient by anointing curcuma anthorhizon or by using roasted lacquer."

In sum, the cure of arthritis and allied conditions was very familiar to Hindu physicians. They had an elaborated system of general, internal, and local treatment, based principally on *alteration* and *elimination.* Apparently they were *successful.*

Greek medicine (treatment of arthritis in the writings of Hippocrates)

If one speaks today about Hippocratism, even to educated physicians who are familiar with the history of medicine, one is told that Hippocrates was a great man indeed and that his merits for the development of medicine in his time were outstanding. His ethic principles are still recognized but his views on clinical pathology and on therapeutics are considered entirely antiquated and useless, like most of the writings of earlier physicians up to a hundred years ago. But this is a grave error.

In Europe the medical profession took a more *positive* attitude towards *Hippocratism*. It had been recognized that his views on the *self-healing power of nature,* and as a consequence his methods of *elimination* such as purging, sweating, vomiting, bleeding, and draining of the skin by counter-irritation are axioms of eternal *lasting value* and must be reanimated to the fullest extent in the light of modern science. The Faculty of Paris, in 1936, founded the "Societé Internationale Néohippocratique" for the purpose of re-introducing Hippocratic thinking and methods into the practice of medicine on a modern basis as the present author has done for many years through his *Constitutional-Therapy*.

In the case of arthritis and allied conditions the Hippocratic methods of *elimination* and draining of the skin are *indispensable* for any effective cure.

Whether the different sections of the Corpus Hippocraticum are genuine or not, they reflect the spirit of that era and have a common background in theory and practice. These writings display an extensive knowledge of arthritis, which is called podagra, and its allied conditions. In fact, acute and chronic gout (which we call podagra today) have in common a metabolic disturbance as a cause. Admittedly the chronic forms especially can be with difficulty separated into the two distinct categories of gout and arthritis.

The *successful cure of arthritis,* except in very advanced stages, seemed to be a matter of course to Hippocrates, and was not burdened with as many reservations as it is today.

Among causative factors Hippocrates recognized the *age* and the *sex factors.* Among the diseases characteristic of old age he quotes: "Distress in breathing, catarrhs with coughing, difficult urination, arthritis, kidney diseases . . . apoplexy . . . itching . . . cataract and deafness" (*Aphorisms* III, 31).

Concerning the influence of the sexual function one reads: "A woman is not taken by podagra (arthritis) before her menstruation has ceased [menopause]" (*Aphorisms* VI, 29).

Modern statistics confirm that 80 per cent of the sufferers of the most widespread form of arthritis, namely osteoarthritis, are women, especially middle-aged women in and after the menopause. If younger women are stricken by osteoarthritis, they usually display too scanty menstruation, producing a retentional toxicosis.

Metabolic disturbances caused by insufficient or absent menstruation are acknowledged by the following quotation: "The wife of a certain Polemarchos who was suffering from pain in the joints, was attacked by a violent pain in the hip, because her menstruation did not appear" (*The Epidemics* V, Ch. 91). On another occasion such arthritic deposits (humoral metastases) disappeared when the menstrual flow was restored to regularity again, which was expressed by Hippocrates with the words: "when she became a woman again."

In the male the influence of the sexual gland is expressed by the well-known sentence: "Eunuchs are taken neither by podagra (arthritis) nor by baldness" (*Aphorisms* VI, 29).

On the other hand, as we shall see later on with Galen, premature gout and arthritis in younger men was known to be provoked often by a dissolute way of life, such as winedrinking and sexual excesses.

In general, Hippocrates reckons arthritis among those diseases that originate from a *superabundance* such as foodstuff, fat, blood, and metabolic waste products. According to the humoral pathology of this epoch, metabolic products are expressed in terms of the four humors. One reads: "Most diseases originate through *bile* and *phlegm*" (*On Internal Diseases,* Ch. 51; See also on Crit. Days, Ch. 8). Another example: "Sciatica may originate from bile but also from phlegm" (*On Internal Dis.*, Ch. 2).

It was also believed at that time (and we may confirm it today), that the majority of all diseases do not come from without, as injury or infection, but from within, and mostly by a surplus of body material, including food and waste products.

"Those who have swellings in the neighborhood of joints or pain as a consequence of fever, take too much food" (*Aphorisms* IV, 45).

"There are three principal causes from which diseases originate, . . . first man falls sick if he is not purged properly." For the two other factors coelestial circumstances (climate, weather, and astronomic constellation, seasons) and injury are quoted (*On Internal Dis.*, Ch. 19).

"To *obesity* and *plethora* obviously, an inflammation of the blood is due to supervene" (*On Diet* I, 35).

Hippocrates described the symptoms of plethora as follows: "With some the whole body aches, with others only one part of the body. . . . In the delusion that they are exhausted, they try to cure themselves by ease [relaxation] and plentiful food, until they run into fever. . . . If, however, fever occurs by neglect, they should take nothing but water for three days. . . . It is also good to use diaphoretic ointments during the crisis, because those expel the disease" (*On Diet* III, 6).

This sentence shows again the disease-producing effect of *overloading the system*. Hippocrates and most of the ancients called plethora not only a surplus of blood, but a superabundance or overfilling of the system in general. This applied also to the treatment of arthritis in overweight, plethoric, and dyscrasic individuals.

Diaphoretic ointments, unknown in our days, consisted in irritant ingredients, such as mustard, resins, etc., and were widely used with good success in antiquity. It would be worthwhile to study them again. We find them also in the medicine of the Hindus.

Another observation, pointing at the salutary effect of *derivation through the skin,* is the following: "In swellings of the joints in infants [rheumatic fever] the eruption of small ulcers [probably pimples or boils] would serve as a cure" (*The Epidemics* VI, 12).

What a prospect is opened by this simple sentence, written more than two thousand years ago! Today, rheumatic fever in children (Still's disease) is one of the most dreaded diseases, crippling human beings for life with heart disease, against which modern medical science seems to be almost helpless, because we hunt after bacteria or virus and adapt our therapy only to this angle.

According to earlier physicians, in such cases antiphlogistic, anti-dyscrasic, revulsive, and eliminatory treatment seems to have been much more promising.

Overcharging of metabolism, or in other words, a corruption or a surplus of the body humors, is a *fundamental cause* of arthritis, rheumatism, and allied conditions, according to the ancients. One reads: "Those in which, as a consequence of fever, lengthy tumors or arthralgias occur, take too much food" (*Aphorisms* VII, 64).

"Sciatica originates from the bile, but also from the blood" (*Crit. Days,* Ch. VIII).

"Those pains in the shoulder that descend down to the hands and cause numbness and pain are not necessarily followed by deposits. Those patients, however, recover if they vomit black bile. . . . This disease [arthritis and rheumatism] in its most violent form attacks men between the ages of forty and sixty years. This stage of life is haunted mostly by sciatica" (*Prognostics* II, Ch. 41).

In the understanding of diseases, especially of arthritis and allied conditions, the conception of humoral metastasis, also called *metaschematism,* plays an important role: "If certain locations of the body take over something from another location, perhaps in the form of pains, numbness, or other symptoms, then it brings recovery" (*The Epidemics* VI, Ch. 23).

The idea of morbid matters circulating in the body and being transposed from one organ to another brought about the methods of derivation and revulsion, drawing pain, inflammation, and morbid matter from vital or important organs to the skin, where the offensive products could be eliminated. This important approach should be revived by modern medicine.

Retention of normal excretions, such as perspiration, bowel movements, urination, hemorrhoidal and menstrual flow may cause a *toxic condition* (autointoxication).

"If menstruation does not flow, women become sick in their system. Why they become sick, I shall discuss in the book on Female Diseases" (*The Semen,* Ch. 40). As the two books on Female Diseases are incomplete, this part, to which Hippocrates refers here, evidently has been lost. However, it shows once more the importance of a regular menstrual flow for feminine health.

"Eliminations according to nature are: bowel movements, urine, sweat, saliva, nasal mucus, menstruation, hemorrhoidal bleeding, outbreaks of the skin, tumors and cancer" (*On Nutrition,* Ch. 17).

The answer to this conception of arthritis as a condition caused by corruption, retention, and surplus of body material, is *artificial elimination* in its different forms, such as purging, vomiting, sweating, bleeding in different ways (venesection and cupping with scarification), also the different forms of draining of the skin by counter-irritation, especially with cauterization.

Evidently all these methods have been *gathered by observation* and especially by watching the self-healing power of nature.

"All diseases originating from overfilling (superabundance) are cured by elimination. All those originating from depletion are cured by repletion. Also the other diseases by their contrary" (*Aphorisms* II, 22).

From this stems the famous sentence "contraria-contrariis," one of the fundamental laws of allopathic medicine still dominating our therapy. The opposite sentence "similia-similibus," which became the fundamental principle of homeopathic medicine also was advocated for certain cases by Hippocrates.

"Concerning people suffering from podagra (arthritis) I have to say the following: Those old people who have had hard swellings around the joints . . . as far as I know, cannot be cured by human art without any exception. They are best cured by accidental dysenteria" (*Prognostics* II, Ch. 8).

In imitation of this experience, artificial, sometimes drastic *laxatives* (e.g. aloes, scammonium, and later on resin of jalap, etc.) were *used successfully* in the cure of arthritis. Also irritant enemas served the same purpose. The old and fundamental sentence: "Qui bene purgat, bene curat" (he who purges well, cures well) holds true also for the cure of arthritis and allied conditions. Hardly any general and lasting therapy can be done in this disease without "cleaning" from the system the metabolic waste products and toxins by purging and other methods of elimination.

Hippocrates and his followers until a hundred years ago distinguished between two principal kinds of purgation through the bowels: first, the purgation downward by laxatives and enemas, and second, the purgation upward by emetics. *Vomiting* from antiquity until a hundred years ago was considered one of the *most powerful* preservatives and weapons against many acute and chronic diseases. Hufeland counted it, together with bleeding and opium, among the three "heroes" or cardinal remedies of medicine. Like purging downward, vomiting not only empties the stomach, the duodenum, and the bile ducts, but also has a far-reaching systemic effect. It is one of the oldest forms of shock treatment, stimulating through the solar plexus the whole nervous system. It also increases the resorptive power of the lymphatic system as very few other remedies do and it has a general "cleaning" effect on the whole system. For this purpose it has also been used successfully throughout the centuries in stubborn cases of arthritis, rheumatism, lumbago, sciatica, and allied conditions. Unfortunately, the understanding of emesis as a fundamental and often indispensable healing method has been lost almost completely in our days, causing unnecessary therapeutic failures in many instances. It should be time to recover this important knowledge.

"Pain above the diaphragm indicates purgation upward (emetics), pain below the diaphragm indicates purgation downward (laxatives)" (*Aphorisms* IV, 18).

This very famous aphorism of Hippocrates, primitive as it sounds, is one of the most *fundamental rules of general treatment* in all medicine, although likewise *forgotten* today. It means that diseases of the head, throat, and chest are often improved or cured by *emetics*, e.g., mental diseases, headache, migraine, tonsillitis, stomatitis, sinus trouble, asthma, bronchitis, suffocation, whooping cough, goiter, laryngitis, pulmonary edema, and pulmonary embolism.

On the other hand, diseases of the abdomen such as gastric atony, diseases of the gallbladder, the spleen, the kidney, the lower intestines, and the female genitalia often can be improved or cured by proper *laxatives,* especially those with chologogue, alterative, emmenagogue, resolvent, or antiphlogistic by-effects. (More examples and case histories proving these statements may be found in the author's textbooks on constitutional-therapy, 1928 and 1953.)

As a rule of general treatment Hippocrates stated the following:

"It is also wholesome to use emetics in order to clean the system, if this has not been achieved sufficiently by physical exercise" (*On Diet,* I, 35).

"If there is a violent pain in the lumbar region (lumbago), even after copious bowel movements, it is beneficial to vomit large amounts of foamy masses by intake of hellebore" (*Coan Prognoses,* 304).

The recommendation of vomiting together with purgation, sweating, and bleeding in the case of arthritis and allied conditions appears frequently in the Hippocratic writings.

Another important procedure in the cure of arthritis, which has also fallen into oblivion, is derivation and *revulsion through the skin* by cupping with scarification and cauterization.

Even Herodotus tells about the savage tribes of the Skythes, at that time populating the steppes of Russia and the Northern Balkans, and how they cured many diseases by creating artificial ulcers through cauterization.

Discussing sciatica Hippocrates also recommended *cauterization* if all the other methods of elimination did not succeed. In antiquity *sciatica* and *coxitis* were not separated distinctly, but treated in the same way, and often enough with success. This sounds rather primitive and incredible, but can be explained for two reasons: first, one and the same metabolic waste product, e.g., uric acid (or in ancient terms "black bile") may settle down on the hip joint as well as on the sciatic nerve. Second, the methods of elimination through bowel movements, vomiting, sweating, cupping, and counter-irritation (cauterization) are equally useful in coxitis as well as in sciatica.

This example, by the way, proves again that practical therapy is often far from congruent with theoretical explanation. Even diseases of still unknown cause can often be cured by established unspecific empirical methods.

Speaking of sciatica (comprising true sciatica and coxitis) Hippocrates said: "This disease originates from the bile but may also originate from phlegm and from the blood, and the pains are similar in all these different kinds of disease". . . (*On Internal Diseases,* Ch. 51). Hippocrates recommended warm compresses, steam baths, purgation with different laxatives according to the supposed causing humor, e.g., berries of mezereum, called Cnidian berries, helleborus, resin of scammonium and of euphorbium.

"If all these remedies do not help, one should cauterize the patient, that is those parts where bones are near to the surface should be burned with *lamp wicks;* the fleshy parts, however, should be cauterized with the *hot iron,* making many deep burns. If, however, the disease originates from the blood, one should prescribe a steam bath, put on a cup and open the veins in the hollow of the knee [fossa poplitea]" (*On Internal Diseases,* Ch. 51).

"If a person is stricken by sciatica, pain occurs in the hip bone [os ischii], in the coccyx bone, and in the buttocks; finally the pain crosses around throughout the whole leg. With such a pain it is indicated to soften the painful parts through bathing, warm compresses, and steaming. Afterwards laxatives must be given. . . . The disease, however, is lengthy and painful, although not fatal. If the pain concentrates on a single spot, remaining there encroached and cannot be expelled by remedies, then the painful spot must be burned with raw flax" (*On Passions,* Ch. 29).

Burning with flax reminds us of Chinese moxibustion, which has been used successfully in such conditions as far back as five thousand years ago.

In the two successive chapters of this book *On Passions* Hippocrates repeated the same recommendation in case of arthritis and podagra, namely purgation, sweating, bleeding and cauterization.

"If the pain of podagra remains in the big toe, one must cauterize the veins of the big toe, somewhat above the joint. The burning should be done with raw flax" (*On Passions,* Chs. 30 and 31).

Hippocrates made extensive and successful use of *cauterization* in all kinds of stubborn or dangerous diseases such as pneumonia, empyema, especially in phthisis and in many diseases of the head (e.g., epilepsy) chest, abdomen, especially liver and in dropsy. He also cauterized cancer, apparently sometimes successfully.

Cauterization of the spine is described in case of spinal atrophy as follows:

"As soon as the patient has put on weight one should burn him in the lumbar region on both sides of the vertebrae with four burns on each side, also on the back, fifteen burns on each side, and on the neck between the sinews two burns on each side. If one is lucky with burning, one may cure the patient."

Another famous sentence advocating cauterization in joint diseases is the following: "If in people suffering from chronic sciatica (mixed up with coxitis) the hip becomes dislocated, then the thigh shrinks (atrophies) and they begin to limp, if they are not treated by cauterization" (*Aphorisms* VI, 60).

Cauterization not only often checks the process of arthritis, but also presents at the same time an effective treatment for dislocation of joints (e.g., the shoulder joint) in producing a shrinkage of the capsule, retaining the end of the bone in its place.

We can find the same extensive use of *cauterization in all Oriental systems of medicine* and also with the primitive nations (Chinese, Japanese, Tibetan, Malayan, Hindu, and Arabian medicine, also with the Red Indians and African tribes). They performed *miracles* by cauterization, which we miss by not using it. Fire has been considered the supreme remedy, superior to all others, expressly by Hindu medicine and by Hippocrates, as is expressed in the following well-known sentence:

"What drugs do not cure, is cured by iron. What iron doesn't cure, is cured by *fire*. What fire doesn't cure, has to be considered incurable" (*Aphorisms* VIII, 6).

Hippocrates stressed (*On Ancient Medicine,* Chs. 1, 2, and 12) that no one can practice medicine without knowing thoroughly the *experiences of earlier physicians.* "He, however, who rejects and despises all that and tries to investigate in another way . . . deceives himself and others."

"I do not claim that one should throw overboard ancient medicine as if it did not exist at all, or that its investigations were wrong, if it is not accurate in every respect . . . but I believe that we have to consult it further and to admire its discoveries which have been made in spite of much ignorance. For beautiful and right are these discoveries and not arbitrary."

In sum we may learn that *arthritis* and allied conditions were considered even by Hippocrates not only a local but a *systemic disease,* probably resulting from a disturbance in the chemical household of the body or in modern terms a metabolic disease. This condition was *treated successfully* by the different methods of alteration and *elimination,* mainly by diet, purging, vomiting, sweating, bleeding (especially cupping with scarification on the painful spot), and finally by cauterization with flax (lamp wicks) or with the hot iron. We shall see that this kind of treatment was followed successfully in a more or less refined way throughout the centuries *until a hundred years ago.*

Greek medicine after Hippocrates

From about 450 until the second century B.C., Greek medicine did not always follow the doctrines of Hippocrates, but sometimes went from one extreme to the other, just as it has in the last two centuries of modern times.

The Dogmatic School (450 to 300 B.C.) tried to fill the gaps left by experience with speculative theories of dogmatic significance, by which the best principles of Hippocrates were abandoned. Chrysippos of Cnidos, for instance, rejection venesection and purgation, two of the main pillars of practical medicine.

The School of Alexandria (300 until 50 B.C.) stressed anatomical and physiological research, but still often overstressed theory first. As a reaction the Empirical School originated in Alexandria. They claimed that only *experience* makes the good physician. The famous "Empirical Tripod of Glaucias" postulates first, personal experience of the physician based on observation. Second, knowledge of the works and experiences of earlier physicians, handed down by historical tradition. Third, conclusions of analogy in new diseases.

The second part, namely the *knowledge of traditional wisdom,* deserves much more attention in our days.

Diocles of Carystos, Praxagoras of Cos, Theophrastus, the famous botanist, Herophilus, Eraisistratus, and Nicandros are the most important names in this period.

It is interesting to know that Pliny the Elder, (A.D. 23-79) criticized severely the dogmatism of the scientific "School Medicine" of his time and stressed empirical folk medicine, as Paracelsus did later.

The treatment of arthritis also was affected by these different schools of thought.

Roman medicine

After a period of empirical, domestic, or home medicine, of which M. Porcius Cato is a well known example, more and more Greek physicians came to Rome.

About the year 100 B.C. they founded the School of the Methodists whose main representatives were Asclepiades and Themison. They overthrew the traditional humoral pathology and replaced it by a more mechanistic solidar pathology, just as Bichat and Virchow did in our time. The established methods of derivation and elimination were abolished and replaced by a kind of naturopathy, consisting of physical therapy, massage, hydrotherapy, etc. All diseases were divided into two categories, namely constriction or relaxation of the pores (status strictus or status laxus). According to the principle contraria contrariis, in the first case relaxing and in the second case tonic treatments and adequate remedies were given. This approach appears to be very exact and scientific, but of course it could not cover the manifold existing morbid conditions. Thus numerous practical methods of healing were lost, just as in our days.

More comprehensive was the encyclopedic textbook on medicine edited by Cornelius Celsus in the first century A.D. In a rather impartial way he summarized medicine from Hippocrates until his own time. He postulated complete knowledge of medical tradition and pleaded against overspecialization ("Ars medica indivisibilis").

In the practical part of his book he also described the treatment of joint diseases as of that time, consisting of different internal remedies, poultices, cupping with scarification and, as the *supreme remedy,* which is still effective even in inveterate cases, he praised *cauterization* with the hot iron.

"Ultimum est, et in veteribus quoque morbis eficacissimum, tribus aut quatuor locis super coxam cutem candentibus ferramentis exulcerare. Sed frictione quoque utendum est, maxime in sole, et eadem die saepius, quo facilius ea, quae coeundo nocuerunt, digerantur. Eaque, si nulla exulceratio est, etiam ipsis coxis, si est, caeteris partibus adhibenda est. Cum vero saepe aliquid exulcerandum candenti ferramento sit, ut materia inutilis evocetur, illud perpetuum est, non, ut primum fieri potest, hujus generis ulcera sanare, sed ea trahere, donec id vitium, cui per haec opitulamur, conquiescat" (*Lib.* IV, *Cap.* XXII). Translated: "The ultimate and even in inveterate diseases the most effective remedy is to cauterize the skin on three or four spots on the hip with the hot iron. Massage also should be used, at best in the sunshine and several times a day, in order to disperse harmful deposits. . . . As there is often the indication to create artificial ulcers by cauterization, in order to make an outlet for harmful morbid matter, these artificial ulcers should not be healed quickly but kept open until the disease has quieted down."

In the chapter "De coxarum morbis" he writes: "Coxis proxima genua sunt, in quibis ipsis non nunquam dolor esse consuevit. In iisdem cataplasmatis cucurbitulisque praesidium est: sicut etiam, cum in humeris, aliisve commissuris dolor aliquis exortus est. Equitare ei, cui genua dolent, inimicissmum omnium est. Omnes autem ejusmodi dolores, ubi inveteraverunt, vix citra ustionem finiuntur." (*Lib.* IV, *Cap.* XXIII).

Translated: "Next to the hip joint are the knees which are also often painful. In such instances poultices and cupping are useful. The same holds true, if pain occurs in the shoulders or other joints. To those who have painful knees, horseback riding is very harmful. Any kind of pain in the joints, if they become inveterate, can hardly be cured without cauterization."

Scribonius Largus

In the first century, before Galen's reformation of medicine, Eclectic Medicine tried to reconcile empirical with scientific medicine and also humoral with solidar and pneumatic medicine. Famous physicians of this period were Archigenes, Rufus, Aretaios, and the outstanding surgeon Antyllos. Among them Scribonius Largus was a very successful practitioner, whose "Prescriptions" (Compositiones) contain important material concerning general medicine and also the treatment of arthritis.

I have used the German translation edited by Dr. W. Schonack, G. Fischer's Verlag, Jena, 1913 (dedicated to Dr. Sudhoff and Dr. Meyer-Steinegg).

Scribonius Largus lived at the time of the Emperors Tiberius (14-37), Caligula (37-41), and Claudius (41-54). His "Compositiones" are the first major comprehensive collection of Roman prescriptions. In the introduction to his book he expounds a few very important principles which we find necessary to quote here: "Herophilus, one of the most outstanding physicians of the past, said that drugs (remedies) have the power of divine hands. For what the touch of a god can achieve is done by drugs which have been tested by frequent use and experience . . . therefore, those should be despised who wish to deprive medicine of drugs. . . . The Ancients treated diseases first with herbs and roots, because the faint-hearted mortals did not easily resort to cutting and burning. . . . Why some people want to discard the use of drugs from medicine, I cannot find out, except that they want to veil their ignorance . . .

"Medicine is the science of healing, not of damaging. If it is not eager in every respect to help the sufferer, then it does not provide the compassion due to man. May those who cannot or will not help the sick, stop deterring others, by refusing to patients the help which can be achieved by powerful drugs. Medicine succors the sick step by step. First it tries to help the weak by planned *diet*. If this does not succeed, then it resorts to the power of *drugs;* because these are stronger and more effective than food. If even then the symptoms do not cease, it forcibly turns to *cutting* and *burning.*"

In blaming the incomplete education of many physicians of his time he said: "Therefore, the necessity of studying has been abolished for everybody. There are some, who not only do not even know the *ancient authors* through which our profession came to perfection, but they even dare to contrive falsehoods about them. For where no choice of persons takes place, but the bad and the good one are taken as equal, there observation and wisdom perish and everyone strives after that, which he can get without any effort and which can bring him just as much reputation and profit. Everybody wants to carry on medicine arbitrarily . . . therefore we claim that many, who know *only part of medicine,* wrongfully have acquired the title of credited physician.

"We, however, have gone the right way from the very beginning and stressed the knowledge of the entire medical science, as far as this is possible for a human being . . . therefore, we carried on carefully the use of drugs, as we daily experienced through it success which was achieved sometimes against any expectation and belief of others."

Those words are still potent *today* because the study of the *classics* is *disregarded* and with it the established *empirical methods.* Also the hyperscientific approach, that is, the urge *to know,* to recognize, to analyze, to explain, and to diagnose too often overpowers the urge *to help* the sick by any means whatever, which should be the primary goal of medicine.

Scribonius Largus based his famous collection of prescriptions on his own experience and that of numerous medical predecessors. He considered *most diseases* such as angina pectoris, asthma, epilepsy, headache, dizziness, herpes zoster, cancer of the breasts, rheuma, renal calculi, neuralgia, and arthritis to be *metabolic disturbances.* He removed them mainly by *purgation* with artfully composed remedies, among which colocynth, boletus laricis (agaricus), aloes, myrrh, opoponax, sagapenum, as well as other resins and spices are preponderant. The most important of these compounds he called "Holy Bitters" (Hiera Pikra) and he told of its miraculous effects, especially in arthritis and allied conditions.

Expressly he distinguished between *arthritis* and *podagra*. "In both kinds of arthritis" the *Holy Bitters* are helpful, also in pains of the spine and the lower back, "because it brings relief instantly by purgation, and it also prevents future discomfort. For, those who apply this remedy are *cured in half the time* they were before."

Reports on the wholesome effect of specific purgatives, eliminating harmful substances, return again and again in the whole history of medicine up to our time. Even today the striking effect of certain patent medicines and nostrums for rheumatism, arthritis, and gout may be explained by this mechanism.

For *external treatment* Scribonius recommended a large number of dispersing and softening plasters consisting of resins and other irritant drugs, and we shall find them again in Galen. But altogether they are not of decisive effect, as they do not produce blisters, rashes, or artificial ulcers.

Poultices of herbal decoctions, flax-seeds, fennel seeds, bean flour, barley, soft cheese, wine with wool fat, oil, vinegar, pitch, saffron, live lime, foamy saltpeter, and others were used extensively. Also bathing in warm sea water or in salt water was praised.

Most interesting is his use of living electric rays, which numbed the pain in the leg by electric shock not only transitorily, but allegedly sometimes even permanently, thus anticipating the different forms of modern electrotherapy (diathermy, short waves, high frequency and X-ray therapy, galvanization and faradization).

Archigenes, who lived before Galen under the emperor Hadrian (117-138) wrote a chapter on sciatica and coxitis, "De ischia sive coxendicum dolore." There he recommends cauterization with hot iron and with the glowing roots of the plants Saponaria and Aristolochia. In case of true sciatica (pain of the sciatic nerve) cauterization was applied on three spots, namely near the hip joint, on the lateral side of the knee, and of the ankle. In case of coxitis cauterization was applied on the most painful spots: "Veteres etiam ustione in ischiaticis usi sunt, tum per cauteres ferreos, igni candefactos, tum per struthii (saponaria) et aristolochiae radices coxae junctura in altum perusta, itemque cruri per intervalla quaedam circa dolentes maxime loco cautere admoto."

Galen

About a hundred years later (129-201) lived Galen, who brought about a progressive renascence of the Hippocratic doctrines and thus dominated medicine for more than a thousand years to come.

In his twenty-volume work (I have used Kuehn's edition) there are more or less detailed quotations on rheumatism and arthritis in more than fifty places in his writings. He distinguishes rather clearly between the *podagra* proper and the chronic *arthritis,* which he calls "morbus arthriticus." He is well acquainted with the changing localization of the rheumatic morbid matter, now in the joints and again in the muscles, tendons, fascia, or nerves. According to him, in feverish arthritis refrigerants, and in chronic conditions "heating" (warming) remedies have to be used.

Today the principle of soothing in acute and stimulating in chronic diseases is still valid.

Podagra proper, according to Galen, concerns mainly the feet, but arthritis all the joints.

Galen explains arthritis and rheumatism on the basis of *humoral pathology* through a preponderance of blood, phlegm, yellow or black bile, according to the individual constitution. He attempts the cure by *elimination* of the harmful substances. The latter, according to him, can be recognized from the coloration of the individual, his eliminations, from the by-symptoms, from experience and from the effect of the applied remedies (ex juvantibus).

Among those diseases that originate from *superabundance* (repletion of the body) of food stuff and metabolic products (morbi qui ex plenitudine oriuntur), he counts (besides sore throat, catarrhs, hemorrhoids, and other bloody discharges), eye diseases, pneumonia, pleurisy and other inflammations and also *joint diseases* ("articulares morbi"). Therefore, he prescribes especially at the onset of the disease, in the case of plethora and superabundance, venesection or cupping with scarification, and in addition *purgation* in different ways.

"Qui articulorum vitiis laborant, tenuem victum injungito." Arthritic patients should live on a *restrictive diet*. Obese patients must reduce.

"Podagram aut arthritidem incipientem, quae nondum circa articulos nodos produxerat, vacuatione prohibimus."

Thus Galen cured joint diseases in the beginning, before knotty deposits formed, by purgation with certain drugs, as he did in many other metabolic conditions.

"Nos equidem multos jam a morbis ita conservamus et incolumes tuemur, qui multos annos antea semper aegrotabant, imo et podagram et arthritim adhoc incipientem per vacuationem multos jam annos fieri prohibuimus" (*Comm. Hippocr. Aph.* LXVII).

Compared with our up-to-date treatment of arthritis, we do not make nearly enough use of the *healing power of purgation*.

Among purgative eliminations Galen also counts the menstrual and the *hemorrhoidal* flow. In analogy to the Hippocratic sentence that a woman as a rule is not stricken by arthritis until her menstruation ceases, Galen says more precisely that a woman who "recte purgetur menstruis," (not only still is menstruating but has a menstrual flow, sufficient in quantity and quality) will not be attacked by podagra or arthritis.

Concerning men having hemorrhoidal bleedings, Galen says in a similar way that they "a morbis immunes vitam transigunt," that they live through a life free of diseases. If, however, the hemorrhoidal bleedings are suppressed they may suffer from the severest diseases. Similar sentences we find repeatedly in the writings of Hippocrates.

Coxitis and *sciatica,* as with other ancient authors, are not clearly distinguished by Galen. Sciatica occasionally (but not always) may originate from a surplus of blood and in this case is quickly cured by venesection near the hollow of the knee or the ankles: "citissime curatur venis circa poplitem aut talos sectis" (*Comm. Hipp. Nat. Hom.* II, 6).

Again and again one reads: "Maximam vim ad effectionis curationem habet totius corporis evacuatio." Translated: "Most powerful in order to achieve a cure is *purgation of the whole body*." For this purpose not only laxatives, bleeding, menstrual and hemorrhoidal flow were considered but also purgation upward, by vomiting.

It goes on thus: "Auxiliantur etiam vomitus ipsis ischiadicis magis utiquam evacuationes infernae per ventrem. Faciendi sunt vomitus in principio ab accepto cibo, postea per vomitoria medicamenta."

Translated: "Patients suffering from sciatica are benefited by *vomiting* even more than by purgation downward. Vomiting should be provoked first by overfilling the stomach, afterwards by emetic drugs."

Earlier physicians used to provoke vomiting by overloading the stomach with large amounts of warm water, decoctions of certain herbs, or mixtures of water with vinegar, honey, and salt. Vomiting then was caused mechanically by tickling the throat with feathers, usually peacock feathers. Vomiting as an effective remedy of certain forms of arthritis and rheumatism has been used ever since, until the beginning of the nineteenth century, e.g., it was still used by Tissot and Hufeland.

As *purgatives in arthritis* and rheumatism, mainly colocynth, aloes, agaricus, colchicum, veratrum, scilla, scammonium, and other purgative resins were used. Veratrum and helleborus acted at the same time as emetics and purgatives. Scilla (squill) often was used in the form of scilla wine. Of colchicum Galen said: "Hermodactilus ad articulos ducit purgando."

Translated: "Hermodactilus (i.e., colchicum) attends to the joints by purgation." Also, irritant enemas e.g., with sea water, salt, vinegar, or mustard often were used successfully, especially in case of lumbago and sciatica.

Galen also mentions an Egyptian herb Lycopersium, whose sharp, bitter sap should be able to remove the most violent pain in arthritis.

General systemic treatment, called "cura generalis," again and again was postulated as a principal requirement.

Pain-soothing remedies such as opium, mandragora, and hyoscyamus internally and externally were given only seldom, in case of emergency. Primarily Galen, like the other ancient physicians, tried to remove the pain by elimination of the harmful substances, which obviously is a more lasting and thorough cure than mere sedation.

According to Galen *rheumatism* has an etiology similar to arthritis, namely harmful and superfluous humors, and therefore requires similar treatment. It settles down more on the *soft parts* and the *inner organs.* With the wrong treatment it may become difficult to cure or even incurable. Galen discusses the most frequent mistakes that may occur in general and local treatment. Among the physicians he distinguishes "dogmatici aut empirici medici" and speaks in favor of the latter who do what reason and experience advise. "Quod ratio et experientia suadet."

That proves how much Galen has been misjudged, in being called a dogmatist and a mere speculative theoretician, aloof from practical results, whose writings are no longer worthwhile studying.

Very important and not sufficiently recognized today are the *"humoral metastases"* of arthritic or rheumatic morbid matter from one organ to another. According to Hippocrates and his followers until one hundred years ago, sometimes mental diseases are cured by the outbreak of a joint disease and vice versa; gouty, rheumatic, or arthritic morbid products may, by wrong treatment, be driven into the brain, the nerves, the eyes, the heart, the lung, the pleura, the liver, the stomach, and the intestines and may there *cause* deposits, inflammations, spasms, pain, palsies and *death.* The neglect of these vital interrelations is one of the reasons why angina pectoris, asthma, high blood pressure, vascular spasms and many other refractory diseases are difficult to handle with our present localistic methods.

The physicians of the eighteenth and the beginning nineteenth century, e.g., Barthez, Hufeland, and Johann Peter Frank were still fully aware of these connections and often enough had better therapeutic results than we have today with all our modern equipment.

True, we speak again today of rheumatic inflammation of the eye or of rheumatic pleurisy, but usually under the supposition that rheumatism is identical with infection, as in the so-called rheumatoid arthritis. By this interpretation the metabolic factor is again overlooked, although salicylates and other sudorifics are applied, which however cannot fully substitute for the whole arsenal of eliminatory methods.

Galen was also very familiar with the reciprocity between rheumatism and catarrh of the mucous membranes. According to him, by wrong treatment of catarrh of the mucous membranes, which he calls "fluxiones," severe diseases may result.

On one occasion he said: "articularis morbus, podagra aut coxendicus ad ventriculum migravit." Translated: "Arthritis, podagra or coxitis has traveled to the stomach."

In order to keep the body healthy and to cure such general conditions as rheumatism and arthritis, Galen in his book *De Sanitate Tuenda* (*On Preservation of Health* or *Preventive Medicine*) said that the four "virtutes naturales" have to be kept in good order. These are: (1) the vis attractix (the power of attraction), (2) the vis retentrix (retention of necessary material in the body), (3) the vis excretrix (the natural secretion and excretion), and (4) the vis alteratrix (the power of alteration). In sum, *general treatment* means regulation and restitution of all natural functions. This is also indispensable in every treatment of arthritis and allied conditions.

Among other pertinent observations the following are interesting: Diseases of the kidneys, podagra and arthritis, etc., "omnes coitu exacerbantur et labuntur in pejus." (All these diseases increase and grow worse by intercourse.)

Before imminent rain, increased pain occurs. He adds to the *diseases of old age,* which finally accompany the old until death, besides diseases of the kidneys, lungs, and heart, also podagra, *arthritis* and sciatica. Bathing and spas were considered to be wholesome.

Other interesting quotations are the following:

"Arthritis solvitur intestini dolore," Arthritis is removed by pain in the intestines; in other words drastic griping purgatives or *irritant enemas* are helpful, especially in coxitis and sciatica. There is a certain analogy between painful derivation through the bowels and counter-irritation to the skin (*Comm. Hipp. Humorib.*, Ch. I).

"Arthritis biliosorum humorum purgatione indiget," Arthritis requires purgation of the bilious humors (*De Purgatione,* Ch. I). In fact, *cholagogue laxatives* such as senna, rhubarb, calomel, jalop, and others have a beneficial systemic effect in many cases of osteoarthritis.

"Arthritis ex plenitudine fit," Arthritis originates from superabundance of body material (*De Sanitate Tuenda L.* V, Ch. 7).

"Arthritis fit ex ciborum corruptione in ventre," Arthritis originates from corruption of the food in the abdomen. This is in conformity with the old saying: "Venter est officina podagrae," The abdomen is the factory of gout, or "Potus, Venus, otium faciunt podagrum," Wine, love, and idleness produce gout (*Ibid.,* VI, 7).

Recent observations confirm that overfeeding, obesity, and plethora may produce uric-acid diathesis, chronic arthritis, rheumatism, neuritis, and allied conditions. It is hard to imagine how such a condition can be cured without the methods of elimination, just by giving vaccines, vitamins, gold injections, or physical therapy.

In general, these conditions are characteristic for the middle-aged and aged. If gout or noninfectious arthritis occurred in younger men, they were considered to be due to a dissolute way of life and therefore looked on as shameful. "Turpe est, virum robustum arthritide laborare" (*Ibid.,* V. 1).

It was considered still more shameful if a physician (especially in his younger years) was stricken by arthritis or podagra. "Medicum eo laborare, turpissimum" (*Comm. Hipp. Epid.* VI, 9).

It is noteworthy that Galen, like all the other authors, considered arthritis, coxitis, and sciatica to be allied conditions with a *common* humoral or *metabolic background,* which therefore require *similar treatment:* "Ischias and podagra morbi ejusdem generis

sunt, et eandem fere postulant curationem" (*De Remed. Parab.*
I, 16).

Modern overspecialization, which tends to stress anatomical and
localistic findings, has torn apart the close connections between
coxitis and sciatica. The same metabolic product may settle down
at the same time or in succession at the joint, the muscles, or
the nerve, thus producing coxitis, lumbago, or sciatica—which indeed respond to similar methods of elimination and derivation.
Still more clearly we can see this on the shoulder joint where
often arthritis, bursitis, muscular rheumatism, and neuritis of the
nerves of the upper arm are combined. All these respond to derivation and elimination.

Galen used a large number of *internal* and *external* remedies in
a way similar to that of Scribonius Largus. Poultices and plasters were used, containing sedatives, and also irritant substances
such as hemlock (cicuta), numerous resins and corrosives such
as quicklime, alum, auripigment (sulfide of arsenic), sulfur, etc.
Galen claimed that such plasters "omnem duritiem emolliunt"
(soften all hardness) and that they absorb all solid swellings
around the joints and free the patient of pain ("collectiones circa
articulos consistentes absorbent et a doloribus liberant").

Galen mentions expressly that they have an especially strong
effect because they made the skin sore, achieve the exudation of
serous body fluids, and even produce blisters.

The more handy vesicants such as cantharides plaster or mustard plaster apparently were not yet at Galen's disposal. Otherwise he would not have had to resort to such complicated con-
coctions as water in which old sharp cheese was boiled with
salted pork. However, Galen claims that with this remedy he was
able to cure patients "who could no longer walk and had to be
brought to him by cart and wagon."

Galen does not often mention cauterization with hot iron, in
contrast to Hippocrates and his followers until Celsus.

Summarizing we may say that *during Antiquity, arthritis,* rheumatism, and allied conditions were *treated very efficiently,* especially by Greek and Roman medicine, and in many respects

even much *better than by us* today. The basic theory that some more or less fluid morbid matters, whether called humors or metabolic waste products or toxins, are the principal cause of arthritis and rheumatism in most cases, is still valid today. Infection, injury, wear and tear are not nearly as important in the majority of such cases. Ancient physicians, therefore, were right to stress "cleaning of the system" by *elimination* and derivation through the bowels and through the skin, the latter by sweating, cupping, and *counter-irritation*.

We shall see that this fundamental conception, won by direct observation and treatment of the sick, was continually upheld, developed, and refined during the following centuries until a hundred years ago, when contact with the established traditional methods was disrupted. If we wish to improve our practical results, which are far from being satisfactory today, we must re-animate the successful methods of earlier medical systems and combine them with modern diagnosis and technic.

Treatment of arthritis during the middle ages

Alexander Trallianus

Characteristic of the early Middle Ages is Alexander Trallianus, a contemporary of the Emperor Justinian in the sixth century. He wrote an extensive textbook on medicine and drew from his own large practical experience, but he also referred to the writings of his predecessors Paulus of Aegina and Aetius of Amida.

He wrote twelve chapters on medicine of which the last one deals with arthritis. I have used the German translation, edited by Theodor Puschmann, Vienna, 1878.

Alexander comprised all kinds of arthritis under the name of podagra and distinguished between an acute and a chronic form of gout. This may seem confusing at first glance, but from a therapeutic standpoint it is more important to stress the common or *similar metabolic background* of *gout* and *osteoarthritis* than to deny such relations and to emphasize mainly the anatomic and pathologic differences.

In his time the disease was considered difficult to cure or even incurable, for different reasons. According to Alexander, one of the principal reasons repeating itself in the course of history was that the ability to judge rightly the different *causing factors* and the different *individualities* of the patients in each case had been lost because of a tendency to oversimplification, localization, pedantry, and overspecialization. For such reasons, Alexander said, "the disease got the bad reputation of being beyond any cure of the medical art. I, however, claim that this disease, if one distinguishes the differences and single forms of it, according to quantity and quality, can be cured easily by the physician."

Today it still makes a great difference in the cure of arthritis whether obesity, plethora, high blood pressure, amenorrhea, natural, premature, or artificial menopause, biliary disfunction, insufficient elimination by the skin, chronic indigestion, constipation, or uric acid diathesis contributes to the underlying factors.

Alexander Trallianus, according to the doctrine of Antiquity, considered disturbances in the balance of the four *humors* (blood, phlegm, yellow bile, and black bile) to be principal causes of arthritis. In the case of arthritis caused by blood or bile (we may speak of sanguineous, plethoric, or biliary temperament) he recommended cooling and soothing remedies, whereas in phlegmatic and melancholic constitutions he used warming and stimulant procedures. He also blamed *improper habits of living* such as abuses in eating, drinking, working, and in sexual relations as well as passions and aggravations such as exaggerated ambition, envy, greed, anger, fear, etc.

Today once more worry and too much physical and mental strain in general are recognized as important causing factors of arthritis and allied conditions.

Alexander used *venesection, leeches,* and *cupping* with scarification in certain forms of arthritis and rheumatism. In the case of middle-aged and aged patients where a tendency of "thickening" of the blood is evident, such procedures are still very helpful, especially in the case of lumbago, backache in general, sciatica, and muscular rheumatism, particularly in plethoric individuals.

Most important were different *purgatives,* compounded carefully in a complicated way, and used according to the constitution of the patient. Such alterative laxatives usually consisted of resins such as scammonium, aloes, colocynth, and of agaricus, elaterium, and colchicum. Bitter tonics, to protect and to strengthen the digestive organs were usually added.

Alexander praised especially the "Vinegar-Mead of Julian" in which also squill, rhubarb, mandragora, asarum, and veratrum were contained. "This also is the medicine which one has to use, if one wishes to be completely freed of the disease."

"Through such procedures the patient will become free of impurities and fluxions in the future, and he will not have to be afraid of attacks of suffocation [this means angina pectoris and asthma caused by transposition of gouty material to heart and lung], nor any other danger."

One hundred years ago the most outstanding physicians, such as Barthez and Hufeland, like most of their contemporaries, still believed that *angina pectoris* and some forms of *bronchial asthma* may be caused by *gouty metabolic products,* causing spasms and deposits in heart and lung. Angina pectoris was even called a "gout attack of the heart." Consequently these earlier physicians successfully cured such dangerous heart and lung conditions by the methods of derivation and elimination, whereas our modern localistic methods often fail.

Like Hippocrates and Galen before him, Alexander also believed that one should consider the *astronomic constellation* while giving medicine. We shall see the same idea also among other physicians during the Middle Ages and the earlier centuries of modern times, especially with Paracelsus. Here, too, the last word has not yet been spoken, as we know that living organisms are subjected to cosmic and astronomic influences. We know something about the influence of the phases of the moon and of the seasons, but concerning many other cosmic influences such as sun spots, the eclipse, and others we may only guess.

Alexander Trallianus also used *external applications* in arthritis extensively. Poultices of fresh and boiled herbs, fats of different animals, and manifold resinous plasters were used.

"I know that the resin euphorbium boiled with oil and wax has removed great pain. . . . Especially such remedies which warm, irritate, and *blister* the skin [e.g., mustard and garlic with vinegar] are promising." In fact, euphorbium is an effective ingredient of many nostrums for arthritis and also mustard, garlic, horseradish, and onion with vinegar are still used today successfully by the folk medicine of different countries.

"I also saw still another one, who in a similar way used *cantharides plaster* and was very grateful for it. When the vesicles, caused by the medicine, burst, much fluid trickled out, after which he felt great relief."

This principle of *draining of the skin,* even recognized and quoted by Galen, is fundamental and *indispensable* in the treatment of arthritis, rheumatism, and allied conditions. This procedure was developed more and more systematically throughout the following centuries with great success, but unfortunately has been *discarded* almost completely *today* through a shift in medical theory.

Another method of treatment was with salves that disperse and resolve the hardening and deposits of the joints. Such ointments mainly contained the resins euphorbium and galbanum, as well as laurel oil, usually combined with different animalic fats. Among them was a remedy which, according to Alexander, "is effective even in deep-rooted conditions, and *cures* even the so-called *ankylosis* [stiffened joints]."

"This remedy is helpful even in palsies and has also an alterative effect on gouty nodes."

A strong counter-irritant under the name of "Indian Powder" possesses a "truly divine power . . . it is also effective in very large swellings, especially those of the knees."

Podagra caused by *plethora* (fullness of blood) was treated by bleeding and restrictive diet. Especially in the spring one should cut down on meat and wine and increase physical exercise, "because abuse of wine drinking is harmful for full-blooded individuals."

Under improper treatment, the harmful substances may flow back from the joints to vital organs, and may cause danger of suffocation or death of the sick. Therefore, besides the local dispersing and resolving treatment, one should always try "to clean the body completely of the impurities."

In contrast to our *up-to-date skepticism,* Alexander describes a case history where "someone who had suffered for a whole year from large knots of the joints, was restored completely by the use of a certain medicine, so that he *could walk again* without any difficulty." This potion consisted of agaricus, gentian, centaurea, valerian, aristolochia, gamander, spikenard, and parsley with honey. Antidyscrasic, alterative, purgative, diuretic, and bitter drugs thus were used in different combinations, according to the patient's constitution.

To *soothe pain* Alexander used warm softening compresses with or without opium, mandragora, and hyoscyamus. These remedies were given also internally in case of necessity, although, according to ancient authors, one should try always first to remove the pain by elimination of the morbid substances. The herb hyoscyamus (henbane) was called "holy herb" by Alexander, because of its outstanding painsoothing power. It is not used enough today.

"Some also drink the so-called 'hermodactylus medicine' (colchicum), whereby they are often relieved immediately of their pain, because manurelike morbid products are eliminated by bowel-movements. Thus the patients are able to walk again right away. This remedy is reliable and seldom has disappointed our expectations."

"As, however, this remedy offends the stomach and upsets the appetite, bitters or spices are always added. The drugs which contain caraway, ginger, and pepper, thus counteracting the stomach-offending effect of the medicine, are excellent. But nothing is as wholesome as the addition of aloes (bitter tonic with laxative effect)."

Today *colchicin* is given in a pure crystallized form, because we believe that this is more exact and scientific. But many patients cannot stand the large doses necessary to be effective, whereas the *skillful compositions* of the past considered these physiologic reactions.

Optimistically, and apparently based on frequent success, Alexander claims: "This medicine liberates the sick from their pains." Or "this remedy restores the faculty of walking immediately." Or "This prescription cures the pains of the legs, the joints, the head, the stomach, the eyes, the liver, and kidneys." This again expresses the possibility of systemic and universal spreading of gout or arthritis in different organs.

Alexander quotes other remedies which by external application were able "to soothe the pain in a miraculous way (e.g. psyllium)."

Different mixtures and pills were recommended as effective: "This also is the medicine which one may use confidently, if one wants to be freed from arthritis completely."

Another remedy "has helped in a marvelous way and prevented a relapse of rheumatism."

"Very promising are those external remedies which warm, irritate, and blister the skin. I know somebody who even during the most violent attacks was freed of the pains by the mere external use of mustard."

Alexander Trallianus characteristically said that he collected many of such *useful remedies from old writings* and that he published them on purpose, "as the average physician, busy with his practice, has not the leisure to read old books."

This is still very true today. "The history of a science is science itself" said Goethe. Other outstanding physicians of the past emphasize that *study of the classics* and *observation of nature* are two *indispensable* fundamentals of medicine. Today erroneously the writings of earlier physicians are often looked on as outmoded and useless and therefore not to be studied at all anymore.

Alexander gives the prescription of "a simple ointment to disperse and resolve the induration of the joints." It consists of euphorbium, oil of poplar, wax, and goosefat.

Another remedy "is effective even in the most stubborn constitutions and deep-rooted disease and cures the so-called anky-loses." It contains different resins such as galbanum, euphorbium, storax, thapsia, turpentine, oil of spruce, oil of laurel, opoponax combined with wax, oil, and fat. Also salt, pepper, and other irritants were used.

Furthermore one reads, "this remedy possesses a truly divine power, effective even in paralysis of the limbs."

Another "excellent salve which removes the knots of the joints so that no sign of a swelling remains" contains a mixture of resins and alkalies.

Alexander Trallianus quotes the irritant poultice of Galen: "The great Galen tells us that he had cured tophi with old cheese, used in the following way: If somebody has knotty arthritis, I take old very sharp cheese, mix it with the suds of salted pork and put it on the joints. By this method I have the best success. The skin breaks open by itself so that one has not to make an incision (scarification with cupping); and quickly and painlessly, day by day, single parts of the knots disappear." Today hardly anybody knows about such procedures. At present the healing power of colchicum has been rediscovered for acute and chronic gout. But it may be useful also in other forms of chronic arthritis. This was well known to the ancients. Modern French medicine used extract of colchicum extensively for different forms of arthritis, rheumatism, uric-acid diathesis, and allied conditions in the form of the well-known patent medicine Liqueur Laville, a mixture making colchicum more agreeable to the stomach.

In stressing proper individualized diet, Alexander Trallianus *discourages milk drinking,* because it makes the blood "slimy." We shall see a similar conception later on with Paracelsus, Syden-ham, and Barthez.

Arabian medicine in the treatment of arthritis and allied conditions

Arabian medicine very often is disposed of with the phrase that it was only a degenerate variety of the medicine of Antiquity.

But closer study proves that such claims are incorrect. First of all historians state that far from the whole original material is known and many of the available textbooks are partly corrupted Latin translations. Furthermore, we should study more fully the Asiatic systems of medicine, such as the Chinese and the Hindu systems, from which Arabian medicine seems to be more influenced than is usually recognized. True, outstanding Arabian physicians such as Avicenna, Rhazes, Avenzoar, Averroes, Mesua, Maimonides, and Abulcasis, who lived between 600 and 1500, based their writings on Hippocrates, Galen, Aetius, Paulus of Aegina, and Alexander Trallianus, but they added a great deal of their own in clinical observation, especially pharmacology (alchemy) and therapeutic methods taken from Persia, Syria, and India.

Arabian physicians followed the classical conception that *arthritis,* podagra, sciatica and allied conditions are essentially *metabolic disturbances,* caused by a surplus or corruption of body humors. Consequently *purgation* of the harmful substances was the principal indication. A large number of laxatives with alterative-, cholagogue-, and phlegm- (mucus) eliminating side-effects were used. Besides the traditional classic remedies, new alchemistic and exotic drugs were introduced. Especially senna and Indian myrobalanes (which eliminate the bile and phlegm, according to the Arabs) were recommended and also certain metallic remedies that later on were adopted by Paracelsus, in spite of his deprecatory judgment of the Arabs.

Diet, hydrotherapy, occasionally using cold water, warm springs, counter-irritants, plasters, and vesicants, were entirely familiar to the Arabs. They claimed that *artificial ulcers* or *blisters* should be kept open until the pain has gone.

Coxitis and *sciatica,* which were still confused, were treated according to similar principles. Cupping with and without scarification was important. Especially effective were enemas with acrid irritant substances: "Ex hoc enim frequenter sanguis provocatus, schiaticos liberavit" (Avicenna). Translated: "In this way often blood was discharged, liberating the sick from sciatic pain." In other words bloody bowel movements after such irritant enemas were especially wholesome. This reminds us of the Hippocratic sentence, that dysenteria may cure the severest forms of arthritis.

Again, according to the experience of the ancients, *vomiting* was considered helpful. One reads: "Ischiadicis conveniunt prae omnibus vomitus." Translated: "Above anything vomiting is wholesome to people suffering from sciatica" (Avicenna).

At that time they believed that vomiting by "purgation upward" may clean the system of harmful substances. Today we know that vomiting stimulates the resorptive power of the lymphatic system, thus removing morbid deposits. At any rate this method of treatment was upheld by the most outstanding physicians until one hundred years ago as very effective and I can confirm this also by my own experience.

On an especially high level with the Arabs were the different forms of *cauterization* with chemicals and with the hot iron. Particularly concerning cauterization with hot iron (ignipuncture) they had very exact rules and indications, derived of long experience, pertaining to form, size, and location of the points of cauterization. As a rule the hot iron was inserted through the whole thickness of the skin. In this way more powerful and lasting effects on the joints can be expected than by the superficial cauterization with moxa or by the "point de feu" of the modern French physicians, not to mention vesicants or chemical caustics.

One may shudder at such reports and may look down at such methods as cruel, outmoded, and superfluous, although many modern operations are much more superfluous (e.g., tonsillectomy in most cases) and more harmful for general health (e.g., hysterectomy in younger women without urgent necessity).

On the other hand, we may read that the Arabian surgeon Abulcasis was able to cure even the most stubborn destructive arthritis of the hands by applying one cauterization over each finger joint and several such burns over the wrist. This should be reason enough to study these methods all over again.

The physiological and pathological laws of these cauterizations with their incontestable, baffling, and often instantaneous healing effects are not understandable at first glance for our (rather crude and mechanical) anatomic and physiologic conceptions. They may be interpreted more plausibly by *reflexotherapy* as they represent the basis of acupuncture and moxibustion of the Chinese with their more "functional anatomy" concerning vascular reflexes and their idea of a special kind of circulation of fluid in the nervous system or their possibly electric nature.

Abulcasis also confirmed the strange claim of Hippocrates, probably taken from Indian medicine, that under certain circumstances *sciatica* could be cured by one single *cauterization* with the hot iron in the region of the basal joint of the *big toe*. (According to another version, between toes 4 and 5.) It reads: "Non cesses ergo facere illud, usque quo perveniat sensus super mediatione usque ad ancham et quiescat dolor." Translated: "Do not cease therefore to do this (cauterize), until the sensation reaches above the joints up to the hip and quiets down the pain." Thus by violent reflex action from the periphery to the center, cauterization was applied until the pain had gone. We may also partly explain the effect by shock.

The external treatment of arthritis and allied conditions in the Middle Ages was carried out to a great extent by *surgeons* through application of softening ointments, irritant dispersing plasters, leeches, cupping with scarification, vesication, and cauterization. According to their numerous case reports they were very successful in treating this disease. Henry de Mondeville, who belonged to the famous university of Montpellier in the thirteenth century, wrote extensively on this subject.

He said that there are always diseases caused by morbid matter that defy all medication and for which *cauterization* is the *ultimate remedy,* according to Rhazes and Abulcasis ("quibus cauteriam est ultimum remedium . . . postquam medicamina omnia defecerunt"). Cauterization also was used to soothe intolerable pain ("maxime si fiat cauterium propter sedationem doloris intolerabilis").

He deplored the fact that only few physicians are surgeons, and on the other hand few surgeons were scientists, therefore the subtle knowledge and art of cauterization as a whole fell into defamation *unjustly,* and had been almost *discarded* entirely by the modernists of that time ("ideo cauteriorum scientia tota immerito diffamatur et fere dimittitur a modernis"). Apparently the highly refined knowledge of cauterization with its numerous delicate rules and indications, as it had been practiced at its best by the Arabs, was in a state of decay at that time.

How much more must we deplore that the whole of this valuable method has been completely *lost to us.*

The scholarly practitioners of internal medicine in the Middle Ages did not like this part of treatment, as they looked down on surgery in general. As is known, they did not even perform venesections themselves, not wanting to stain their hands with blood. This was one of the reasons why *barber surgeons* and *military surgeons* developed rather independently from scientific medicine. They were less handicapped by scientific *dogmatism,* and also kept in closer contact with the populace and with folk medicine. Thus they rose to increasing significance. The *empirical medicine* of these wound surgeons and even of lay healers, collecting important knowledge just on the difficult subject of arthritis and rheumatism, developed quietly and independently. This wisdom, collected by coincidence, observation, and traditional experience was adopted into their systems by such men as Paracelsus and Ambroise Paré.

Modern times

Paracelsus

At the threshold of the modern age stands Paracelsus, the archrebel of medicine, who also brought about a big change in the cure of arthritis and allied conditions. He embraced all *arthritic* and rheumatic conditions under the name of "tartaric diseases." The word "tartar" comes from the Greek word for wine sediment. Paracelsus believed that harmful *metabolic products* were precipitated in the human system in a fashion similar to the tartar in a wine barrel. There was an added significance in that the name Tartarus was the symbolic expression for the Greek underworld, since the morbid "tartaric" deposits could cause "infernal pain."

The analogy goes still further in that Paracelsus successfully treated tartaric diseases with the *salts of tartaric acid* (e.g., potassium tartrate) just as we use today for this purpose other tartaric compounds such as Rochelle salt or Seidlitz powder. Paracelsus thus followed his doctrine of signatures, based on the laws of similarity, anticipating the second Hippocratic principle: similia similibus, which was later on adopted by homeopathy.

As Dr. Sigerist pointed out clearly in his oration on Paracelsus (in commemoration of Paracelsus' four hundredth birthday), the discovery of America as a new world coincided with a general struggle against petrified authority in many walks of life. In medicine too the doctrine of the ancients had degenerated into rigid dogmatism, appearing very accurate and exact, but becoming more and more remote from the practical truth and therefore often meeting with therapeutic failure, whereas a more natural approach would have been more effective.

It was Paracelsus who protested violently against this *hyperscientific attitude*. (We need such a man just as much today). On his long journeys throughout the whole of Europe, from Turkey to Sweden and from France to Poland, he collected not only the teachings of the medical schools of physicians of *different nations*, but also the knowledge of the *alchemists*, as well as that of the simple folks and *lay healers* such as herbalists, barbers, gypsies, shepherds, hangmen, quacks, and so on.

The result was an entirely different kind of medicine, very often performing apparent *miracle cures* to the amazement of other physicians, whose official dogmatic medicine had failed.

One of Paracelsus' greatest achievements was the successful treatment of arthritis, which at that time was considered nearly incurable, or at least difficult to cure, just as in our days.

The greatness of a physician also may be partly judged by his finding of simple truths that are valid for many instances. Not only "pushing slowly forward step by step intricate and narrowly limited detail work" by overspecialization, as is the ideal of our time, but also crystallizing of *elucidating principles* and effective general treatment of the patient as a whole, are necessary. Such guiding principles can often be won better by unprejudiced free observation of nature on the living organism itself than by artificially intruding the dead auxiliary sciences of the laboratory (that is physics and chemistry) alone.

One of these enlightening principles, especially concerning arthritis, pronounced for the first time in the history of medicine, is surprising in its simplicity and range:

"Where nature produces *pain,* there it accumulates *morbid substances* and want to *eliminate* them. If nature does not succeed by itself in this purpose, the physician must make an artificial outlet (blisters, cupping, cauterization, etc.), right on the sick spot and thus cure quickly the pain and inflammation."

This sentence is one of the fundamentals for a successful cure of arthritis and allied conditions, but it is hardly known or used at all today, which explains the shortcomings of the usual routine in this field.

In many cases in which we today think of infection and localized or mechanical causes, Paracelsus blamed a *disturbed metabolism.* He did not fully subscribe to the view, current even today, that gouty and arthritic deposits are largely constitutional, hereditary, degenerative, or due to aging, wear, and tear, and therefore incurable. His was an *optimistic* view, induced, no doubt, by his own remarkable successes. His contemporaries, with whom he was forever battling, falsely held that joint diseases, marked by permanent swelling, were incurable.

The Roman poet Ovid wrote the well-known line: "Nescit medicus nodosam curare podagram." "No physician alive can cure the knotty arthritis." Paracelsus paraphrased the verse by substituting the word "rhoeades," tyro or would-be physician, for medicus. The inscription on his tombstone at Salzburg reads: "Here lies the famous Doctor Paracelsus who was able to cure with marvelous art and skill such dire plagues as leprosy, podagra, dropsy, and other incurable diseases."

The *treatment of arthritis* according to Paracelsus was performed in *three ways:* first, internal treatment by resolving alteratives, and *elimination* of these mobilized products by bowels and kidneys.

Second, external treatment of the diseased joints by *mollifying* ointments and plasters. These consisted of a mixture of resins and different kinds of animal fats, e.g., resin of euphorbium and turpentine with the fat of dogs, marmots, and badgers. Different oils such as those of laurel, poppy, and muscat were also used. This was called the "closed" external treatment and was supposed to soften the deposits and to take away the stiffness, making the joints flexible once more.

Paracelsus called arthritic deposits "grains." "They must be resolved by drugs," he wrote, "so that they become soft as honey or spun sugar, until the hardened or crippled joints may again be stretched, become soft, and regain their former aspect." No other medical author has so graphically and optimistically described the healing processes in arthritis.

The third kind of treatment was the so-called "open" method, consisting of *draining the skin* by vesication or artificial blisters, artificial rashes, and artificial ulcers caused by chemical or vegetable corrosives. In extremely stubborn cases cauterization with the red-hot iron supervened. Cupping with and without scarification and sometimes leeches also belong to this form of treatment.

Evidently all three of these fundamental methods are almost completely forgotten and *discarded today,* which again explains the frequent failure of our present-day routine. Paracelsus commanded a huge variety of drugs and methods for treating arthritis, and so he was able to perform "miraculous cures" impossible to others. This is still feasible today, if we follow his advice as this author has done for many years, after having studied, translated, and edited the writings of Paracelsus into modern language.

Paracelsus prescribed strong *vegetable extracts* in the treatment of gout and arthritis to be taken in meat broth or wine, believing that they need a "swift vehicle" to penetrate into the blood stream immediately. His theory was supported by his success. That reminds us of the prescriptions of Scribonius Largus and Alexander Trallianus, who added bitter tonics to their vegetable antiarthritic drugs (e.g., colchicum), in order to protect the stomach from being hurt by these rather acrid substances. Meat broth and wine act in the same way. To this day French medicine, as quoted above, successfully uses certain herb wines against gout and arthritis—the famous Liqueur Laville is an example.

In addition to plant remedies, Paracelsus knew a large number of *mineral* and *chemical drugs* with "resolvent" effects. Preparations of *mercury* and *antimony* particularly enabled him to achieve astonishing cures similar to those achieved with *gold* injections today. Moreover, he and his followers successfully used a complicated organic compound of colloidal gold for the cure of arthritis, which apparently was harmless, whereas modern injections with gold admittedly are still risky and sometimes even dangerous.

Tartar emetic (tartrate of antimony), today likewise almost forgotten in spite of its manifold curative powers, was at that time ascribed such miraculous effects that one spoke of "Antimony's Triumphal Vehicle," as the title of a contemporary book on the subject. It was likened to Cerberus (cerberus triceps), the triple-headed hound of the underworld, because of its threefold power to cause vomiting, purging, and sweating.

Moreover, tartar emetic in small subnauseous doses (e.g., 0.01) has a strong resolvent, antiphlogistic, resorptive, dispersing, mobilizing, and alterative power. In a similar way, mild preparations of mercury such as *calomel,* likewise in the smallest doses, are extremely useful especially in decreasing the swelling of the soft parts in osteoarthritis.

Vast experience and unusual success caused Paracelsus to fight violently *against the pessimism* concerning arthritis in his time.

"Who has filled you with such madness and despair," he cried out, "as to believe that there is neither drug nor relief for podagra?" He bade the Emperor to stay the learned schools with their falsehoods from barring his new method of treatment, based on age-old experience.

"I have achieved cures that were not possible for the physicians with all their books." (*Paramirum,* Huser, Vol. II) "Arcanum, that means to restore someone against all the rules of the physicians."

Such plaintive notes are again timely in an age in which traditional experience is once again forced into hiding before modern dogma . . . the exaggerated and misinterpreted dogma of "exact natural science."

Only recently (1942) an American medical authority, Dr. Alan Gregg, director of research at the Rockefeller Foundation in

New York, in a lecture on "Medicine and Humanism" delivered at the New York Academy of Medicine, stated that just as medicine, in dealing with the living man, once had to defend itself from misguided theology, so now it must fight against the "dead hand" of exaggerated natural science, that is, physics and chemistry.

Paracelsus mercilessly castigated the single-track specialists. "The divided doctors," he said, "are the disrupters of medicine. The one can do this, the other that, but in none of them is there true wisdom. For he who knows only a piece of it knows nothing, nor does he know what he can do." (II. *Book on Podagra,* Huser, Vol. II).

This is especially true concerning arthritis. It cannot be treated by the orthopedist, physiotherapist, endocrinologist, or surgeon alone, except as all these combine the knowledge of an efficient practitioner in internal medicine and surgery in order to take care of the manifold causes and sources of arthritis, especially the most widespread form, osteoarthritis. Treatment of the *patient as a whole* is hardly anywhere as necessary as in the *cure of arthritis*.

Paracelsus wrote several books and treatises on arthritis and allied conditions which, as mentioned before, he called "tartaric diseases." He comprised in this clinical entity all kinds of deposits in different organs, just as in the nineteenth century the French spoke of *arthritisme* and other clinicians of *uric-acid diathesis*.

Renal calculi, gallstones, calcification of the arteries and of the heart, ossification of the inner ear, causing deafness, deposits in the eyes such as cataract and glaucoma, etc., were grouped under this common denominator, and treated successfully by similar methods of resolution and elimination.

Here, too, a more general and broadminded approach opens more favorable aspects for successful treatment than does pedantic overspecialization.

Many other *challenging statements* about arthritis were uttered by Paracelsus: "Five mysteria and arcana which resolve the podagric tartarus are known to me . . . all of them are resins. Through those salves the tartaric grains are resolved, which otherwise cannot be dispersed."

Among the numerous *vegetable drugs* given by mouth as resolvent medicine is herba gratiolae, called "Herb of Mercy of God," *Gottesgnadenkraut* by European folk medicine, because of its strong alterative resolvent, emmenagogue, and laxative power. Together with colchicum it is still a main ingredient of many nostrums for arthritis and gout, usually extracted in wine.

In contrast to our *up-to-date skepticism* ("there is no cure for arthritis") toward historical and empirical knowledge, Paracelsus upheld a decisive active *optimism in therapy,* which manifested itself in many characteristic aphorisms:

"This powder cures all rheumas and fluxions, and all tartaric diseases by resolving the stones . . . as water disperses tartar or another salt" (*Ueber Steinkrankheiten, Huser,* Vol. II).

"Through this remedy every podagra, chiragra, and similar diseases can be cured."

"In this way you can expel every podagra by force." That concerns the application of artificial ulcers.

"Those medicines which we have quoted now, are able to cure every contracted joint" (*Ueber Contracturen der Glieder, Huser,* Vol. II).

"In tartarus, there is a special power, because it possesses the property to penetrate the whole body, and it is especially helpful in palsies" (*Ibid*).

"He who wishes to cure podagra, must act as indicated by microcosmic anatomy." That means correct interpretation of symptoms.

"If this should be achieved, it requires minor surgery, such as artificial ulcers, cauterization, bleeding, etc." (*Podagric Diseases,* Huser, Vol. II).

"I am writing on podagra, which until now has not been described truly, and has not been cured by any physician.

"I do not speak only of podagra, but also of all other diseases, about which they do not get any word of the truth. What decent and good things can you expect, if hangmen, knackers, monks, nuns, etc., excel them in it, and occupy themselves too with medicine. . . . Emperor wake up! If you do not turn the tide when you should, the murder will be permanent" (*Podagric Diseases,* Huser, Vol. II).

These are embittered outbursts of a representative of liberal-minded *empirical medicine* against the opposition of the *dogmatic school*.

"There are three things, which are required to a complete cure of podagra: purgation, opening of the skin and furthermore specific treatment" (*Ueber Podagra,* Huser, Vol. III).

"Threefold is the way of healing and it restores health of that which is mutilated and crippled . . . the way of expelling the disease is new, and it is in contrast to the books of the physicians."

Paracelsus also counted cerebral hemorrhage or *apoplexy* among the tartaric diseases. He called it *gutta* which means drop, probably signifying the drop of blood discharged into the brain. The French word *goute* which means gout is a further link in the chain of these connections. Paracelsus, like many other earlier physicians, prevented and treated apoplexy and other symptoms of arteriosclerosis with antiarthritic, alterative, and eliminatory remedies, in a much more active way than that of up-to-date clinical routine.

One of the *most enlightening* quotations in all the writings of Paracelsus is the following, partly quoted already above: "If you find somewhere *pain* at any location, you should know that nature wants to have an outlet on this spot. If it is not there by nature, then make one yourself, because nature wants to have it here and nature hurries only towards the outlet . . . therefore look to it to be ready *to make an outlet* ("emunctorium"), as it corresponds actually to the circumstances, or by another way through corrosives, as in podagra, sciatica, arthritis, etc. For it is almost one third of the whole of medicine that a physician should know how to direct the expulsive power (of nature), according to its will." (*Comment on Hippocr. Aphor;* Huser, Vol. II).

Only occasionally Paracelsus refers to praiseworthy predecessors: e.g.: "I shall describe the cure of podagra, according to the best masters of medicine."

"Arcana for colic and contractures are hidden in the fats and oils." That refers to the oil-and-glycerine-cure of gallstones and renal calculi and to the intensive application of different kinds of fat in joint diseases.

Even Hippocrates, who has been quoted as the highest medical ideal, is considered by Paracelsus as deficient in many respects, because he did not yet possess alchemistic knowledge. Podagra cannot be cured without alchemy, according to Paracelsus "for the seeking has been with him, but the gift of the end (perfection) was not given to him, and therefore Hippocrates died before (the arrival of) art. Art is long, life however is short" (*Ibid*).

Paracelsus also deplores the helplessness of the Chaldean and Arabic physicians concerning podagra and stony deposits.

In order to overcome the resistance of the *dogmatic medical schools* he often appealed to high ranking persons; for instance:

"Therefore attention, you chiragric lords and you podagric princes, why do you have to suffer more severely than the lower class people? Listen carefully to our writings . . . you will learn from them that there is a possible cure, although this has been denied by the oldtime teachers and their followers."

There is considerable truth in this outburst, as high-ranking people as a rule go through the whole machinery of scientific tests and treatment based on the latest fashionable unproved therapy, whereas the plain people, especially out in the country, more often stick to established simple natural and traditional methods, usually frowned at by the medical schools.

In *"stone diseases"* Paracelsus distinguishes between an *internal* and a *surgical treatment*. Concerning internal treatment he quotes two kinds of remedies: "One kind breaks the stone. The other kind consumes and dissolves the salt." A large number of such drugs are quoted as simple or compounded recipes (Huser, Vol. II). We may learn from it that Paracelsus (like many other physicians until a hundred years ago), in contrast to the up-to-date pessimistic conception, considered renal calculi and gallstones to be soluble. Stone is transformed into gravel and is eliminated that way.

In his book *On the Contractures of the Limbs* (Huser, Vol. II) the different causes of stiffening arthritis are discussed extensively such as injury, stone deposits, repressed abdominal colics, anger with consequent biliary disturbances, habitual drinking of certain stone-forming wines, etc.

He enumerates a group of alchemistic remedies such as Essentia

Antimonii, Oleum Vitrioli, Arcanum Sulfuris, Aqua Tartari, and others, which one reads: "We have named here remedies, which were not known to the ancient physicians. . . . Those remedies which we have mentioned now, are able to cure every contracture."

Another book *On Podagric Diseases and Related Conditions* (Huser, Vol. II) begins with the words: "Therefore I am willing to write on podagra, which has not yet been described truthfully or cured by any physician. They babbled a lot, but few deeds were achieved."

Much of it applies to the one-track-minded overspecialization that often ignores the necessary interrelations with the organism as a whole, e.g., the frequent origin of arthritis, but also of diseases of the skin, eye, ear, and nerves from the abdominal organs of metabolism.

One of the *written consultations* of Paracelsus, still handed down (Huser, Vol. II) recommends certain laxative candies (lozenges) and venesection as a protection against apoplexy and podagra: "This regime protects against podagra and deprives it of its violence and malignancy . . . it prevents and consumes the podagra so that it cannot move and come on for many years."

A certain herbal wine is recommended by the following words: "That will consume the fluxions in your head, and also in the joints where they are lying."

"Four things you should avoid: strong flavored wines, rich food, anger, and women. The more abstemious you are in these things, the better for you."

In the *Opus Paramirum* (Huser, Vol. I) Paracelsus delivers a long treatise on the origin of all diseases from the Tartarus. As such he understands tartarlike deposits in the body that are due to improperly chosen or badly worked up food, "With all the old rules one cannot achieve anything here, because they all have never understood the resolution of the tartarus and still don't understand it today. Therefore in this field they harvest only shame and disgrace, and soon kill the patients with their prescriptions."

Paracelsus also emphasizes the liver in connection with tartaric diseases: "For the *liver* is the *root of many diseases*. It is a vital organ on which many, nay, almost all organs depend."

In fact, we may trace biliary diseases in the history of many arthritic patients. Also, tartaric salts are known as beneficial to osteoarthritis as well as to liver and gall bladder conditions.

Again and again Paracelsus turns *against* these physicians who indulge mostly in dialectic verbalization and *theoretical explanations:* "They grow up in the medical school only as babblers and scribblers." . . . "Who writes prescriptions (and as for today— who makes only diagnoses) but doesn't heal anybody, is nothing but a scribbler, and therefore only a doctor of writing but not of medicine."

Very drastically he describes how the *tartaric,* we would say the arthritic-rheumatic morbid *matter,* may provoke conditions of irritation in entirely different organs, such as *spasms* in the heart and the stomach, spasms in the bronchial muscles (asthma, colics in the kidney and gall bladder, apoplexy, etc.).

Dissolution and elimination of the tartarus, according to Paracelsus, may also cure organic diseases. Not only by way of the bowels through purgatives, but also through the skin, such morbid products may be eliminated: "For the sweat is the excrement of the blood." . . . "These are the finest excrements, the result of the "third digestion" which exists in the whole body. . . . The sweat however is visible and palpable although it was before in a gas like condition in the system" (Huser, Vol I).

This corresponds to the true conception of the vital importance of visible and *invisible perspiration.*

"All joint—and hip diseases, insofar as they are not podagra, are nothing but tartaric fluids (humors), which lie in the limbs, in the nerves of the hip, and in the ligaments, etc., as a fatty sap, causing attacks. He who knows how to treat the stone correctly, may also cure this disease, and he who does not understand the former, is unable to take care of the latter" (*Ibid*).

We wish to comment that very often lumbago, sciatica, and even the beginning of coxitis and other joint diseases may consist in an accumulation of irritant metabolic products. Before lasting deposits are formed they can be easily removed by the methods of elimination.

"From this, it follows, that there are many existing remedies which dissolve, melt, and *break down* such *stones* to clay and flour. For in the stones originally, this condition has been solid. For the solidity of the stone is not so strong that it could resist a remedy whose resolving power is so great" (*Ibid*).

In another book *On Tartaric Diseases* Paracelsus gives an explanation for the name "Tartarus": "Tartarus it is named therefore, because it delivers an oil, a water, tincture, and a salt, that lightens and burns the sick like the fire of hell, for tartarus is hell."

"There are many tartaric diseases in man which are mistaken for other diseases . . . therefore they cannot be cured. . . . From this error and ignorance it follows that they say, it is an incurable disease."

"If a physician wants to protect someone from the tartaric diseases, he must manage first, that the stomach consumes everything that comes into it, just as fire consumes wood."

That means that a *good* functioning of the *stomach* is *important* for prevention and treatment of arthritism.

Interesting is the following sentence: "The ancients *forbade milk* in tartaric diseases, because it is constipating." By that is understood not only constipation of the bowels but also the blockade of the lymphatic vessels by improper metabolic products. For similar reasons legumes such as dried beans, peas, and lentils were strictly forbidden. Many forms of up-to-date and originally well-intended restrictive diets, especially dairy products, oil, certain vegetables, raw diet, and abstinence of meat often do not agree with the stomach and therefore deteriorate the primary disease of arthritis. For similar reasons Paracelsus recommends carbonated mineral waters, in order to strengthen the stomach at the same time. He praises as especially wholesome the springs of St. Moritz, in the Canton of Engadin in Switzerland.

Ambroise Paré

In spite of all the new discoveries in the field of anatomy and physiology made at the same time (Vesal, Falloppio, Serveto) Paracelsus still remained the greatest practicing physician of the first half of the sixteenth century. Concerning our subject, of special importance besides other surgeons of that time is Ambroise Paré, who lived in the second half of the sixteenth century.

In his two-volume textbook on medicine he devotes a large chapter of about fifty pages to arthritis, calling it "maladie ar-thritique—vulgairement appelée goute." He considers acute and *chronic gout* (including arthritis) as a unity that may appear in quite a number of different forms, caused by a variety in constitu-tion, causing factors, and localization. He supposed an acrid "virus," originating through *abnormal metabolic processes* that may receive a special feature by the addition of surplus cardinal humors (blood, phlegm, bile, and black bile) and therefore re-quires different methods of treatment.

Furthermore "There are as many species and differences of ar-thritis as there are joints," therefore the different names podagra, chiragra, gonagra, rachisagra, omagra, sciatica, etc. In the case of too great superabundance of harmful body humors all the joints may be involved.

The names fluxion, rheumatism, catarrh, and arthritis have been invented "because the expression gout is odious, especially to young people" ("parceque le nom de goute est odieux, princi-palement aux jeunes gens").

Reasoning on the "hidden causes" of gout has led Ambroise Paré to the conception that a *metabolic product,* unknown at that time, was in play, which never produces suppuration, but on the other hand causes more violent pain than any other morbid matter, even that of exulcerated cancer. It produces in the joints some-times heat and sometimes cold. The morbid matter is considered so violent and malignant that it may cause under certain circum-stances sudden death (by retrogression into inner organs as in heart attack or brain stroke). The virus is so violent that like the bite of venomous animals it acts more by its quality than by its quantity.

Paré illustrated his experiences with dramatic case histories.

One day, King Francis II's personal physician called him to the Paris court to consult with other physicians concerning the case of a forty-year-old lady-in-waiting who was suffering dreadful attacks in the region of her left hip. Every possible means of soothing the pains had been tried. Many physicians and surgeons and even sorcerers had been consulted—all in vain. Paré applied a corrosive to the painful spot. When the scab dropped off, an acrid dark secretion issued, and from that time on the patient was free of her pain. Like Paracelsus, Paré concluded that he was dealing with noxious substances that escaped when an *outlet* was provided.

A similar incident occurred with the wife of the royal coachman who suffered from such violent pains in her right arm that she was nearly driven to jumping out the window. She begged the court physicians Castellan and Chapelin, as well as Paré, to help her. After consulting with one another, the three physicians created a fontanella (*artificial ulcer*) on the painful spot "et l'ouverture faite, sa douleur cessa, et elle l'a depuis du toute perdue"—once the opening was made, the pain disappeared and never came back.

Of true inherited gout Paré said that it was "like the income from a trust fund, for it appeared each year at definite times, generally the spring and fall."

Paré distinguished between three main causes: hereditary disposition, surplus body humors, and *suppression of habitual secretions* (such as perspiration, menstruation, hemorrhoidal bleeding). Diarrhea and vomiting are also sometimes of importance and must be allowed to run their course.

Illuminating is Paré's insight into the fact that podagra often arises when the body is insufficiently purged of toxins after severe attacks of disease, especially infectious conditions. This basic observation has been forgotten, although it may lead to prevention of many complications that follow in the wake of such diseases as influenza, measles, or typhoid.

In general, earlier physicians did not proceed as nihilistically and expectatively as we do today in the course of infectious diseases. They watched the symptoms carefully and tried to prevent complications such as diseases of the heart, the lungs, the brain, the gallbladder, the nerves, veins, and the joints. They did so by the methods of derivation and elimination. Especially at the end of infectious diseases they urged proper individualized purgation in different ways, in order to "clean the system" of toxins, and afterward they prescribed tonics in order to strengthen and to build up the body again.

Paré was gifted with a typically French sense of humor that in no way detracted from the seriousness of his observations. "Gout sufferers," he wrote on one occasion, "are able to predict weather changes—rain, snow, storm, and sleet—as though they carried a farmer's almanac."

According to Paré, too intensive physical and mental strain may lead to arthritis by impairment of the saps of life and of the metabolic processes. The *liver,* as the largest metabolic gland, plays a central role in arthritis. As we know today, uric acid and bile, the two most important offenders, are produced in the liver.

Arthritis, and especially gout, are reckoned among the most painful and even unbearable diseases, so that "the sick often lose their mind and prefer death instead of suffering any longer." According to Paré the disease is most painful with persons of choleric temperament. In such individuals more often palsies, distress in breathing, gangrene, and sudden death occur. We may confirm that *dark-complexioned individuals* with their more concentrated acrid blood and irritant body fluids may suffer more heavily from gout and arthritis, for the same reason that cancer families (families in which cancer is hereditary) are usually dark complexioned, especially black haired. Intuitively the ancients spoke of a surplus of "melancholia" or "black bile" as a morbid factor in such individuals, and in spite of their vague ideas they were essentially right, as far as the morbid disposition of such individuals is concerned.

Following the tradition of Hippocrates and Galen, Paré believed that women are not subjected to gout (chronic arthritis) as long as they have a regular menstruation, "because by it their whole system is purged" ("tout leur corps se purge"). If *menstruation stops* too early, he continues, many humors and materias (waste products) accumulate in the body which often *provoke arthritis*.

My associates and I can confirm this on the basis of many hundreds of patients, that younger women suffering from arthritis usually display too scanty or too rare menstruation with or without simultaneous obesity and plethora.

For a successful cure, according to Paré, in a way similar to that stated earlier by Alexander Trallianus, the recognition of the *special constitution* is necessary. With sanguinic and plethoric patients, for instance, sparse diet, external and internal antiphlogistic remedies, also general and local withdrawal of blood are necessary. With phlegmatic and lymphatic individuals, on the other hand, warming, roborant, and dispersing remedies are required. With choleric individuals, who are supposed to have a hot and dry constitution, according to the principle: contraria-contrariis, cooling and moistening remedies are indicated. Also *purgation* and vomiting often are recommended for such individuals. In the case of the melancholic temperament, similar procedures were undertaken, but relief of the portal venous circulation by *bleeding the hemorrhoidal veins* was especially considered.

This piece of knowledge also has fallen into complete oblivion today. Draining off the system by menstrual and hemorrhoidal flow, according to long observation, was supposed to rid "the factory of many morbid products," that is, the abdominal circulation, from harmful substances. How naïve, clumsy, and primitive in comparison does our up-to-date routine appear, using one-track specific medicines such as vaccines or vitamins.

Paré mentions that the ancient physicians preferred *vomiting* to all other kinds of purgation in treating arthritis. He also gives explanations for this fact, on the ground of humoral pathology. This may be wrong, but, what is more important, the procedure itself is in practice most effective, because it stimulates all secretions and excretions, as well as the resorptive power of the lymphatic system.

He tells the story of a nobleman in Geneva who for a long time had suffered from a violent pain on his left shoulder so that he hardly could use his arm. The patient had already been treated by different physicians and surgeons. Purgation, venesection, diet, decoctions of guajac and other drugs, as well as different local treatments, apparently salves and blisters, had been applied without any result. Paré prescribed vomiting, but as the patient told him that he could vomit only with greatest difficulty, Paré advised him to have a heavy supper, consisting of different kinds of meat with garlic and onion. He also should drink as much as possible of sweet and sour wines mixed. In the morning he should provoke vomiting with a feather or his finger. This should be done three days in succession. The patient recovered quickly, regaining the free use of his arm. ("Et par ainsi fut du tout guari, s'aidant autant bien de son bras que jamais avoit fait.")

Again and again Paré stressed that on account of the different causing factors, temperaments, and constitutions, *arthritis cannot be cured by a single specific* as is believed by common people ("les vulgaires") and by empirics, who try to cure with one and the same remedy all kinds of arthritis. (Compare the modern oversimplified treatment with gold injections, vaccines, vitamins or cortisone only.)

Paré described a large number of recipes, consisting mostly of *purgatives* with different side-effects, such as cholagogue, and alterative "blood purifying" qualities, among them aloes, colocynth, scammonium, agaricus, rhubarb, senna, hellebore, and colchicum. One of these numerous compositions bore the name "pilulae arthriticae."

According to Paré the law of medicine consists mainly of addition and subtraction, and as arthritis originates mostly through superabundance of humors, purgation and bleeding have been found extremely useful. "There are no better remedes than those."

The toxin of arthritis may penetrate elsewhere, causing extreme pains "and asking only to find an exit out of the system, therefore one must open the door (il faut ouvrir la porte) in whatever form it may be, such as by application of cups, scarification, vesicants or cauterization."

Among *local applications* those plasters and poultices were most esteemed, which make the skin sore and induce the draining (leaking) of fluid serum.

As the most powerful remedy Paré, too, praises the red-hot iron, especially in refractory cases of arthritis of the hip, which at that time still was confused with lumbago and sciatica, although the effective treatment of these three conditions was and still is the same.

In contrast to exaggerated localization and subdivision of the different forms of arthritis, rheumatism, and allied conditions, Paré like most of the ancients knew that one and the same harmful morbid product may attack not only the joints but also the muscles, nerves, blood vessels, the heart, lung, stomach, eye, ear, and other organs. Therefore general internal or *systemic treatment* was considered *indispensable* in arthritis.

Paré also described *muscular spasms* in the neck, the arms, and the legs on the basis of gout, recommending proper habits of living, sufficient exercise, as well as dispersing and eliminating internal and external remedies.

Today the interpretation of such cramps in the neck and in the calves has had to be rediscovered and uric acid had to be traced as a cause. If today we call those cramps in the calves "intermittent cludication" we rather think of local arteriosclerotic processes, often forgetting the common metabolic cause such as arthritis or uric-acid diathesis, which of course blocks the way to successful therapy.

The other surgeons of the sixteenth century were like Ambroise Paré also eager not only to be specialists of *surgical technic,* but to understand the so-called surgical diseases as much as possible from the *internal angle* and to treat them accordingly either by themselves that way, or with the help of the scholarly physicians. Therefore we find such treatises in almost every major textbook of this time; e.g., with Fabricus Hildanus, Percy, Minderer, Dionis, etc. Everywhere careful treatment of the metabolism of the body humors and also intensive local treatment including vesication, fontanellas, and cauterization were applied and proved as established.

Modern surgery has discarded most of this and only now is again beginning to consider temperament, general health, and constitution of the patient, whereas counter-irritaton is still neglected.

◆

The problem of arthritis in the seventeenth century

The seventeenth century was an era similar to ours, in which *natural science* was the ruling principle in medicine. The iatromathematic, iatrophysic, and iatrochemical schools bore their names from such tendencies. In many respects the new discoveries of natural science brought *progress* and enlightenment. But on the other hand modern historians of medicine admit that by precipitating an exaggerated application of these principles, *many errors* were committed, and in *discarding* the established *empirical methods* of the past frequent failure in treating the sick occurred.

We have little to change in such statements and the analogy to our times can be recognized.

Among the iatrophysical school Santorio and Baglivi, among the iatrochemical school Sylvius, were best known. They applied the doctrine of the acid and alkaline "acrimonias" of the blood in the interpretation of arthritis. Especially important, however, was the understanding of the significance of invisible perspiration in the origin, prevention, and cure of rheumatism and arthritis.

Santorio proved by exact experiments that the human body eliminates daily about two pounds of waste products by invisible perspiration, consisting of water damp, carbon dioxide, and volatile organic acids. He and his follows until the beginning of the nineteenth century and including Hufeland, reasoned that qualitative or quantitative inhibition of this vital process of elimination may cause *a retentional toxicosis* or autointoxication, by accumulation of irritant acrid waste products, which may cause congestion, pain, inflammation, and deposits in different organs such as joints, nerves, muscles, tendons, and also in the eyes (rheumatic iritis), in the lung (rheumatic pleurisy), and even in the brain and spinal cord, causing there inflammation and degeneration whose etiology, without this obvious supposition, is still considered unknown and enigmatous. This working hypothesis was and still is so valuable in practical medicine that it deserves much more consideration than it is given today.

The therapeutic answer to this interpretation is the extensive application of *perspiration* as a basic healing method.

Sylvius, for instance, said that "one third of all diseases may be cured by proper perspiration," just as many other diseases can be cured by proper purging (qui bene purgat, bene curat). This is also the deeper purpose of hydrotherapy, which stimulates not only the circulation in the skin, but also the eliminatory function, that is, invisible perspiration.

Sweating and invisible perspiration can be promoted not only by exercise, *hydrotherapy*, air, and sunbathing, *steam baths,* and sweating cabinets, but transitorily and permanently by a certain group of *drugs,* called sudorifics, among which not only the salicylates but also small doses of tartar emetic, acetic ammonia (Minderer's spirit), ipecacuanha combined with opium (Dover's powder), and many vegetable drugs, such as tiliae flowers, elder blossoms and, strongest of all, the leaves of jaborandi with their crystallized product pilocarpine, are important.

In the seventeenth century, metallic preparations of *gold, silver, mercury,* and *antimony* were favored by another group of physicians who were exponents of alchemy, also in successful cures of arthritis. Poterius, Zacutus Lusitanus, and others published their case histories in so-called "centurias," that is chapters of one hundred cases each. Often these observations were called "praxis admiranda," which means miraculous cures in severe or stubborn diseases. Among them many cures of severe arthritis were reported.

In his book, *Opera Omnia Practica et Chymica,* Poterius repeatedly writes: "remedium eficacissimum in arthritide est aurum diaphoreticum," "The most effective remedy in arthritis is sudorific gold." This is a complicated, apparently colloidal compound of gold, combined with organic substances, so that it was less offensive than the inorganic compounds and could be given by mouth in effective doses without any harm.

Poterius describes a number of cases of acute and chronic *arthritis* and also gout, which he cured mainly *with* his famous compound of *gold.* He says expressly: "The radical cure of podagra consists mainly of diaphoretic gold" ("radicalis podagrae cura consistit maxime in aurum diaphoreticum"). Furthermore, he says "that for this disease ordinary remedies are not enough, but they must be taken from the realm of metals." . . . "Mercury alloyed with gold (mercurius fixatus cum auro) is nothing but diaphoretic gold. . . . By setting in motion strongly the flow of lymph this remedy removes all obstructions excellently." . . .

In stubborn cases sometimes preparations of *mercury* alone were given successfully, until salivation occurred, according to the great seventeenth-century physician Wedel ("Salivatio mercuralis rite instituta feliciter tollit podagram"). Salivation is accompanied by excitation of all secretions and excretions together with an increased resorptive power of the lymphatic system.

One reads (*Centuria Prima,* pp. 19-21): "Pulvis antipodagricus est aurum diaphoreticum." . . . "est aurum cum mercurio junctum."

The following paragraph is a comment made by the great Frederick Hoffman, who edited and commented on the work of Poterius.

"Memini olim tali medicamento mercurialis inveteratam podagram tophosam sanatam in sexagenario Halensi, ita ut per plures annos firma usus fuerit valetudine." "I remember that sometime ago with this medicine, I cured a sixty-year-old man from Halle (Germany), who had suffered from an inveterate knotty podagra so that he could enjoy a number of years further in good health."

Poterius himself, among other case histories telling of successful cures of arthritis, described a case of severe arthritis of the knee and hip that had been somewhat improved by extract of hellebore and of colchicum: "dato tandem pulvere nostro antipodagrico ad 5. vel 6. dies tantum . . . cito et jucunde convaluit." "Finally having taken our antipodagric powder for five or six days only, he recovered quickly and easily."

Other outstanding physicians called mercury *"the tamer of rheumatism."*

It was also in the seventeenth century that the Dutch physician Tulpius discovered (or rather rediscovered) that *arthritis* is often *cured* quickly and surprisingly if the patient happens to break out with smallpox, itch, hives, or other *skin eruptions*. He recognized this effect as being nature's way of draining the toxins out of the sick spot and from it he learned the value of artificial rashes and blisters in curing arthritic pain, stiffness, and deposits.

As a matter of fact, this knowledge of the striking healing powers of *counter-irritation* was familiar even to the primitive nations in prehistoric times.

Tulpius in this connection made a few more important observations. He said: "Look at nature, you surgeon! As if it were a finger, it points at the wholesome use of artificial ulcers . . . they are useful in arthritis, they expel soreness of the eye, but nowhere are they more useful than in epilepsy" (Tulpius, *Observationes Medicae,* Lib. I, Cap. 8).

One of the most outstanding physicians of the seventeenth century was Sydenham, called the "English Hippocrates." Although he was no academic teacher at any medical school, but just a simple practitioner, he won such an international reputation that his epitaph reads "Medicus in omne aevum nobilis"—a physician excelling through eternity. He became famous for his amazing practical success in numerous cases in which the usual scientific routine of his era failed. As in our time, the collected practical experience of the past was overruled by the newly rediscovered natural sciences, such as mathematics, physics, and chemistry. Sydenham on the other hand followed the established tradition in the form of a progressive Hippocratism. In chronic diseases he stressed the *elimination* of undigested and superfluous humors and the strengthening of the stomach and of the metabolism. In the case of arthritis or gout "the whole constitution has to be altered and the individual, so to say, freshly rebuilt."

He was a virtuoso in using the simple fundamental methods of healing such as purgation with different drugs, vomiting, sweating, and bleeding.

Concerning diet he emphasized that one should not take more food than the stomach can digest. On the other hand the organs should not be weakened by too great abstinence. The taste of the patient should be considered, as very often that which the stomach craves for is digested quicker, even though it may be heavier than bland food which does not agree with the stomach. Very significantly he stated that *milk diet,* in spite of some advantages, agrees very badly with many persons. Moreover, it suppresses and *weakens all normal functions* because of a lack of stimulus. Pure water, too, if taken in large amounts, is considered harmful, because it may produce gastric atony. According to him light beer, which is more tasty and stimulating, as well as small amounts of Spanish wine, are preferable.

In overfed and arthritic individuals transitory restrictive diet consisting of whey was recommended, and also preparations of ammonia (e.g., acetic ammonia) in Spanish wine, night and morning, and a fontanella (artificial ulcer) on the leg, in order to drain out morbid substances. A "blood purifying" potion protecting at the same time from renal calculi consisted of a decoction of sarsaparilla, sassafras, root of cinchona, and hartshorn salt, sweetened with licorice and anise. This potion had to be taken over a long period. For arthritic and gouty people horseback riding also was advised, "because it stimulates the metabolism as very few other things do."

In the case of dangerous *regression of gouty material to vital organs,* e.g., the heart, lungs, or brain, opium alone or in combination with camphor was given as a lifesaving remedy, provoking hyperemia of the skin and critical sweat.

Summarizing, we may say that there is definite evidence that the physicians of the seventeenth century were very often able to *cure* different forms of *arthritis more effectively than we do today.*

Eighteenth and beginning Nineteenth Centuries

In this era we find humoral pathology at the height of its flowering, enriched by the new discoveries of physics and chemistry, refined by highly developed philosophical and clinical thinking, and supported by a profound comprehensive knowledge of practical historical facts unknown to our generation.

The treatment of arthritis, rheumatism, and allied conditions, too, was on a high universal level and in the hands of prominent physicians, as well as those of well-trained practitioners, yielded healing results from which we can only learn in humble admiration.

In the writings of Boerhave, van Swieten, Hoffman, Stahl, Tissot, Hufeland, Stoll, de Haen, Wichmann, Weickardt, Selle, Vogel, Barthez, Pouteau, Rust, Chelius, and many others we still can find a gold mine of information concerning effective methods of treatment, confirmed by numerous records of successful cures.

These physicians distinguished clearly between genuine gout and *chronic arthritis,* which was also called arthritis anomala. They were well informed about the relation of external and internal rheumatism to the catarrhal diseases. They also knew that there are intermediate (transitory) forms in all these conditions, which today gradually reappear coyly under new names and disguises, and are often enough hailed as new discoveries.

They knew much more about the regression of rheumatic symptoms from external organs to vital inner organs such as heart, lung, pleura, brain, spinal cord, nerves, eyes, and ears, causing there pain, inflammation, deposits, palsies, thromboses, embolism, and other dangerous and even fatal conditions.

The expression *"rheumatism,"* derived from the Greek word *rheuma,* from *rhein,* flowing, (just as the word *catarrh* is derived from the Greek word katarrhein, flowing downward) is based on the supposition that accumulated fluid morbid matters flow about in the system and that they may settle down in all the organs. Rheumatism of the external organs involves mainly the muscles, joints, ligaments, and bones. Rheumatism of the inner organs concerns the organs of the chest, the eyes, ears, brain, and nerves. Even today the expressions rheumatic pleurisy, rheumatic heart disease, and rheumatic iritis are customary, but the interpretation has changed so that nowadays the adjective "rheumatic" means infectious, whereas the humoral pathologic interpretation, meaning *irritant metabolic products,* has been discarded, erroneously, we believe.

Some years ago, Eppinger and Maresch in Vienna spoke of *serous inflammation* on the basis of well founded and numerous autopsies and laboratory experiments, confirming the humoral conception of earlier physicians. This humoral interpretation provides the great advantage of immediately effective therapy, consisting of elimination by bowels and draining of the skin, whereas the infectious interpretation is not only doubtful but rather blocks the way to effective therapy, and leads to pessimism.

As in the seventeenth century, one believed in the significance of the function of the skin as an etiologic factor for arthritis and rheumatism. If the *eliminatory function of the skin* becomes impaired in quantitative or qualitative respect, then acid and acrid metabolic products are retained in the body, called at that time "serum acre retentum," causing all the symptoms of arthritis and rheumatism.

As chronic arthritis often originates as an aftermath of *acute articular rheumatism,* it is worthwhile to look at the great difference of approach to this condition now and then. Acute articular rheumatism was considered a "hypersthenic inflammation of the blood," and not an infectious disease. Even today the infectious origin has not been established beyond all doubt. The disease is not contagious, and a specific virus has not been found. Consequently, these earlier physicians treated acute articular rheumatism successfully with *antiphlogistic* remedies and methods such as venesection, leeches, saltpeter, small doses of tartar emetic, tartaric salts in general, ammonium chloride, ammonium acetate, and vesicants. A large number of sudorifics also was available, but often was considered contraindicated in certain constitutions, whereas today sweating by salicylates is used uniformly and almost as the only valid method in this condition.

Today the complication of *heart disease* in acute articular rheumatism is considered an almost inevitable feature in a high percentage (up to 60 per cent) of cases. In these earlier times, however, purposeful and often successful prevention was attempted. Whenever the symptoms of congestion, oppression, and pain in the chest occurred, our medical predecessors applied intensively the methods of derivation and revulsion such as leeches in the region of the heart, cantharides plaster, venesection, calomel, digitalis, and antiphlogistic mineralic acids, etc. It was almost considered the result of malpractice, if heart failure developed.

In a similar way, an effort was made to prevent metastases in the kidneys and the nervous system, in contrast to our present more "expectative" and fatalistic approach.

According to eighteenth-century physicians the disposition to *chronic rheumatism* is favored by all kinds of weakness of different organs and functions, such as skin, digestive organs, gallbladder conditions, metabolic disturbances such as obesity and "dyscrasia," disorders of the portal circulation, menstrual disturbances, menopause, etc.

As another source of chronic rheumatism, neglected feverish diseases were considered, such as acute rheumatism (rheumatic fever), measles, scarlatina, influenza. Our medical predecessors stressed purging the system of toxins after infectious diseases by the methods of elimination, especially purging, sweating, and bleeding. Afterward tonics were given, in order to strengthen the body.

The treatment of chronic arthritis or rheumatism consisted mainly in *stimulation of all secretions and excretions,* especially of the skin, bowels, and kidneys; also intensive *counter-irritation* was applied as an almost indispensable help. A large number of alterative, resolvent, antidyscrasic, and also specific antirheumatic and antiarthritic drugs were available, such as resin of guajac, aconite, colchicum, herba gratiolae, tartaric salts, mercury, and antimony.

Very characteristic of the eighteenth century is the *Enchiridium Medicum* by Johannes Kaempf, edited by Dr. Kortum in Frankfurt, 1792. Kaempf, a court physician to the Grand Duke of Hesse (Germany), became famous for his method of treating successfully many diseases by a variety of medicated enemas. They were known under the name of "Kaempf's Klystiere." Dr. Kortum, a practicing physician and poet, won a lasting place in the history of literature as the creator of the comic epos, "Die Jobsiade," a satiric student's *roman* in verses.

The *Enchiridium Medicum,* a booklet of 244 pages in a small format, comprises in a very concise aphoristic form the whole of internal medicine. The statements and observations on arthritis and rheumatism are made with such certainty that they must have been established by long and successful experience.

Internally, they took care of the different types of constitutions and instituted first a proper general treatment. Moreover, purgation, sweating, vomiting, local and general bleeding were considered a matter of course. As alterative antiphlogistic and antidyscrasic remedies, tartaric salts, especially Seignette salt and tartar emetic, were recommended, also other preparations of mercury and antimony, especially antimonium crudum, and "soap of antimony."

Externally mustard plasters, vesicants, moxae, cupping, and artificial ulcers were applied. The original text written in laconic Latin sentences enhances the impression of precision and established truthful experiences.

One of the most comprehensive monographs on gout and arthritis in this era was written by P. I. Barthez, professor at the University of Montpellier. He discussed this subject from all possible angles and gave a complete catalogue of all effective remedies (*Traité des Maladies Goutteuses,* par P. I. Barthez. Paris, 1802).

Barthez claimed that in *gout* and *arthritis,* which he considered to be *related conditions,* there is a specific morbid quality of the *fluid parts* of the body. "This specific alteration of the fluid parts can be doubted only by those who are blind enough to exclude from their medical system the diseases of the saps or the humoral pathology completely."

In a very broadminded way he said that one and the same disease can be treated successfully according to very different methods. This should be heeded by those modern authors who want to cut down the treatment if possible to one or two stream-lined specific methods.

In acute articular rheumatism it is most important to remove the inflammatory fluxion by general revulsive and derivative or local bleeding, according to the rules for the treatment of fluxions. Only after that, other revulsive methods such as purgation and sweating are permitted, but always in accordance with the patient's constitution. Also local counter-irritation is required.

He believed that asthma and *angina pectoris* are usually caused by a *rheumatic-gouty* matter. "If these causes of spasmodic asthma are very violent, then they may produce the disease, which the English (Heberden) call angina pectoris, whose paroxysms may hamper circulation and respiration instantaneously and thus may cause sudden death." Consequently he treated angina pectoris like rheumatic pleurisy with local bleeding, vesication, and opium combined with other antispasmodic drugs such as camphor, asafoetida, and ipecacuanha. The latter combination, called in modern pharmacopeas Dover's powder, is still one of the best existing remedies for the most painful attacks of angina pectoris, sometimes of much better and more lasting effect than morphine, or than nitroglycerine, as I have found out myself in a number of cases, and as it was advocated by many outstanding physicians of the eighteenth and nineteenth centuries.

Since our present results in treating angina pectoris and coronary thrombosis are far from satisfactory (every day the newspapers report men dying from these conditions at the early age of forty-five to fifty-five) in spite of the best available medical care, we should consider the humoral interpretation of this condition and try the adequate antispasmodic, revulsive, and eliminatory treatments.

Barthez also gives a history of the treatment of arthritis, quoting the healing methods of many other earlier physicians. Among others he quoted the German physician Trampel, who claimed to have cured several patients, crippled and maimed completely by gout, through the use of cinchona extract and *setons*. The latter are still used successfully by veterinarians in different countries.

A large number of vegetable and mineral alterative drugs are recommended on the basis of established experience, among them decoctions of the sprigs of spruce, dulcamara, and the root of *burdock,* as well as resin of *guajac* dissolved in rum.

As another specificum in gout and chronic rheumatism, a winy decoction of lycopodium, is praised by Lange. A special Decoctum antipodagricum was prescribed by the Pharmacopoea of Vienna at that time.

The textbooks of pharmacology at that time contained a special group of *antiarthritic* and *antirheumatic remedies,* among them resin of guajac, aconite, cicuta, camphor, volatile compounds of ammonia, the root of saponaria, and senega.

The great Boerhave recommended as often wholesome in the most deep-seated forms of arthritis, pills of *medical soap* (sapo medicatus or Castile soap), which according to him one could take for a whole year without any harmful consequence. The dose is 1.5 Gm. three times daily. Other authors of that time also claimed that there is no more effective remedy in arthritis than soap, as it is the most powerful resolvent of the gouty matter. *Radix saponariae* is credited with a similar effect: "Resolvit spissitudinem arthriticam," it dissolves the arthritic thickness in the system.

The authors of that time were familiar with and saw the best results of all kinds of *counter-irritation* such as cupping, leeches, vesicants, moxae, artificial rashes and ulcers.

Stoerk, professor at the University of Vienna at that time, is said to have cured repeatedly the most stubborn and inveterate arthritic pains by creating blisters and artificial ulcers with the fresh leaves of *ranunculus*. Chesneau tells us about a man who had been bedridden for three years because of podagra and unable to walk at all, and who was cured by the leaves of ranunculus, applied to the most painful spots.

Another example of the importance of derivation and elimination in arthritis is Boerhave's observation that those who have sweating feet are protected from podagra.

Musgrave, another physician of the eighteenth century, recommended coffee after dinner, claiming that in the French colonies of America and in Turkey where coffee is a main beverage, gout and stone are almost unknown.

Barry believed that a pure vegetarian *diet* is the least fitting for gouty (arthritic) constitutions, because even in a state of health vegetable food is assimilated only with difficulty by the animalic humors. But the truth of this was doubted by Barthez.

Scot called that diet the best which, followed in moderation, produces after each meal a general feeling of gentle warmth in the abdominal intestines, and at the same time serenity and contentment of mind.

Mead, Grant, Werlhof, Zimmermann, and Barthez himself claimed that *milk* in general is *unfit for arthritic patients*. In contrast to the present-day conception, milk agrees only with those who have a strong stomach and take a lot of exercise. On the other hand, it is contraindicated in all persons who are inclined to weakness of the stomach and to cramps. "Consequently there are many contraindications to a milk diet, which forbid its use in arthritic patients. One of the most frequent contraindications against milk is a hypochondriac condition. In these cases the improperly digested milk weakens the organs of digestion, causing fermentation and flatulence." If it later transgresses "the second ways" (that is the lymphatic vessels) it may cause "obstructions of the intestines and other serious evils."

We have quoted only a small portion of the numerous surprising and enlightening views of Barthez and his contemporaries on general medicine and arthritis. We may conclude from those remarks how much *wider,* more colorful and flexible the *approach of earlier physicians* was to our problem, and how much we can *learn from them* in theory and practice.

Hufeland, one of the most outstanding eclectic clinicians of that time, also wrote extensively in his *Encheiridium Medicum* (1812-1832, 6th edition 1836) on arthritis and rheumatism. He was a professor at the University of Jena, at that time personal physician to Goethe and later on director of the famous Charité Clinic in Berlin. His views on arthritis were also very universal and extremely *optimistic.* He considered all possible kinds of *internal treatment,* but also believed strongly in energetic *counter-irritation.* He said: "Great is the power of vesicants and artificial ulcers. They are able to overcome the most stubborn arthritis and even contractures and ankyloses." There can be no doubt that a physician of such high ethical and scientific standards as Hufeland spoke the truth. This should be reason enough to study the writings of such earlier physicians and not to brush them aside as "old-fashioned" and useless.

In this era, too, *angina pectoris,* certain cases of *bronchial asthma,* as well as apoplexy were considered to be *gouty attacks* of these inner organs and were prevented and cured successfully with the methods of derivation and elimination.

As a special variety of rheumatism, *sciatica* (ischias nervosa) was described by Cotunnius in 1783. According to the constitution of the patient, venesection, leeches, cupping with scarification, vesicants, fontanellas, moxae, and setons were applied. Internally ammonium chloride, acetic ammonia, and aconite in increasing doses were prescribed, with a decoction of guajac at bedtime, in order to provoke perspiration. In very stubborn cases cauterization with the hot iron was applied.

Very significant is the statement that chronic rheumatism and arthritis may be caused not only by colds (refrigeration) but also by *repulsed* and falsely treated *skin rashes,* by *suppressed sweat* of the armpits, the feet, and by *suppressed menstruation.* Today we often ridicule such views, but erroneously.

Morbidly increased venosity (that which the ancients called "morbus atrabiliaris") characterized by hemorrhoids, plethora abdominalis, varicose veins, may provide a disposition to rheumatism and arthritis and requires alkaline mineral waters, resolvents, etc.

Lymphatic habitus likewise may create a disposition to rheumatism, and in such cases antilymphatica and antiscrofulosa must be applied.

In this era, too, the prevention and treatment of arthritic or gouty metastases to inner organs (apoplexy, high blood pressure, angina pectoris, coronary thrombosis, cataract, glaucoma, deafness, vascular spasms, renal calculi, gallstones, palsies) played a great role. Reinvestigation of these humoral pathologic methods enables us to solve many such problems, which seem refractory to our more analytic, overspecialized, and experimental approach.

In those times when the housing conditions for the majority of the population were very poor, *tuberculosis of the joints* was much more widespread than today. They treated it successfully with antiscrofula remedies such as *mercury* and *antimony.* Externally *cauterization* with the hot iron improved and shortened the healing result in a way that we hardly can imagine today.

As is known, tuberculosis of the knee or hip joint and of the spine (fungus and caries) are considered today to be extremely lengthy and difficult to cure. Rest in bed or in a plaster cast, sunshine, X rays, codliver oil, vitamins, and good food are almost all that can be done at present. Such cures are supposed to take many months and usually even several years.

I still remember that at the Surgical Clinics at the University of Vienna during the first decade of our century, such tuberculous knee joints were resected, or sometimes even subjected to amputation.

One hundred years ago surgeons such as Rust, Chelius, and Pott in England cauterized these chronic flabby and spongelike swellings of the joints with the red-hot iron and very often achieved a definite cure in a few weeks or months. They claimed, according to the very old medical saying, that *fire* is the *supreme remedy* and that cauterization with the hot iron more than anything else stimulates the power of restoration in the organism, in a way similar to shock.

Rust, who was a military surgeon in Vienna one hundred years ago, wrote a monograph on this subject and among other records, told the story of a youngster suffering from tuberculous arthritis of the knee joint. He needed to be cauterized, but was afraid of the operation. He finally consented because the doctor had promised him that he would be able to attend the performance of a theatrical play in a week, being free of pain at that time. The doctor was able to fulfil his promise.

The famous English surgeon Pott, after whom tuberculosis of the spine has been named *Malum Pottii,* strongly recommended deep *cauterization* on the sick spot of the spine as the quickest and safest cure possible within a few weeks or months, whereas modern expectative treatment takes several years.

It is regrettable that this method has hardly been tried at all by modern surgeons.

Another very convincing contribution to the effectiveness of counter-irritation in *arthritis* and *tuberculosis* of the *spine* is the monograph: *Observations on the Symptoms and Treatment of the Diseased Spine* (more particularly relating to the incipient stages) by Thomas Copeland, London, 1815. Copeland refers to the previous therapeutic success of Pott and other contemporaneous physicians, in treating diseases of the spine with *cauterization* by the hot iron and by chemical caustics producing fontanellas (issues) or artificial ulcers. His case histories concerning such cures are definitely convincing and are a challenge to modern physicians to imitate them.

My own case histories concerning patients suffering from arthritis of the spine, who had defied the customary treatment and had been declared to be hopeless cases and who were freed of complaints by constitutional therapy in a short time, confirm the claims of our medical predecessors.

Decline of our power to heal arthritis during the last one hundred years

With the shift of medical theory from humoral to solidar and cellular pathology, the influence of morbid anatomy and experimental physiology prevailed so much over the collected experience of the past that almost the whole conception on clinical etiology and the established *empirical therapy* of arthritis and allied conditions was thrown *overboard*. Theoretical skepticism and therapeutic nihilism developed increasingly, and today the *prognosis* of arthritis has become unnecessarily cautious and often enough even *pessimistic*.

It was not until fifty years ago that rheumatism was looked upon with suspicion as an unwelcome intruder into the realm of pathology. Thus the famous Viennese orthopedist Professor Adolf Lorenz declared muscular rheumatism as a disease "in which nothing can be tested in the living, and still less in autopsy." Therefore, such a condition was of no interest to a serious scientist and so was left to lay healers and quacks. Another well-known European clinician called chronic rheumatism "a medical laziness in thinking," and a hideout for different diseases which, under this denomination, evade diagnosis and treatment.

Dr. P. Schober (Stuttgart) wrote on the basis of fifty years' experience that during all the time he was a student in Berlin, Tuebingen, and Strassburg, he never saw a case of chronic rheumatism demonstrated in the clinic. Later when he went to Paris in the eighties, chronic rheumatism there was the center of interest. Bazin had originated the doctrine of *arthritisme,* used in the sense of a metabolic disturbance as being the common cause of arthritis and allied conditions. Later on this conception was exaggerated and thus lost part of its original value.

In connection with the doctrine of arthritism in France, the conception of *hepatism* developed, which stresses the well-known interrelation between arthritis and biliary disturbances. We may recall and confirm here again the ancient idea that dark-complexioned individuals with biliary habitus have a greater disposition to severe forms of arthritis and also to gallstones and renal calculi, and therefore require special cholagogue and resolvent "blood thinning" treatment.

In Central Europe the conception of *uric-acid diathesis* as a common etiologic factor for arthritic and allied conditions came to the fore. During the second half of the nineteenth and the beginning of the twentieth centuries the most important clinicians of this era shared this view. To name only a few, Nothnagel, Senator, v. Leyden, Sahli, v. Noorden, Neusser, Ortner, v. Struempell, Haig, and in America Osler represented this theory. Not only genuine acute gout (uric arthritis) but also the chronic forms of gout and of articular rheumatism were explained by a superabundance of uric acid. It was supposed that uric acid or a similar irritant metabolic product of still unknown composition may produce aseptic endogenous inflammations in all possible organs, that is, not only arthritis, but also neuritis, pleurisy, iritis, skin diseases such as shingles, as well as biliary or renal colics.

In practice, however, most of these authors restricted themselves to the prescription of a diet low in purin and of drinking the mineral waters of such spas as Carlsbad, Vichy, etc.

Compounds of salicylic acid and analgetics (antipyrin, amidopyrin) were also applied. Moreover, certain salts of tartaric or citric acid such as uricedin and citarin, as well as the synthetic product piperazin, were supposed to resolve arthritic deposits. Physical therapy and bathing in hot springs completed the regime. But the results achieved with this medication were unsatisfactory.

With the growing tendency to be exact and accurate at any cost, even this conception of *uric-acid diathesis,* which at least as a working hypothesis provided a common background to and a better understanding of arthritis and allied conditions, was discarded because uric acid could not be traced in chronic arthritis. But even in the case of acute genuine gout, a surplus of uric acid often enough could not be found by chemical analysis of blood, urine, and tissues. This very fact should make us more cautious, realizing that far from all clinical symptoms can be traced by chemical analysis or other tests.

With the *abolition* of the *metabolic theory* of arthritis the *treatment* became still more *ineffective,* even though the presence of a still unknown irritant metabolic product is obvious.

Another reason for the *decline* of successful treatment of arthritis was the mounting influence of *bacteriology.* During the third and fourth decade of our century the large majority of authors believed in infection as the foremost cause of arthritis, e.g., Umber, Gudzent, J. Bauer, E. Freund, Veil, Klinge, W. Berger, and in America also a number of outstanding physicians.

Umber (Berlin) especially introduced the conception of "Infect-Arthritis" into the classification of this morbid complex.

As a consequence, the doctrine of focal infection, supposedly as the most frequent cause of chronic arthritis, prevailed. Tonsils and suspicious teeth were removed on a large scale. Gradually we are realizing now that this factor has been greatly overestimated.

But still the dominating tendency is to believe only in a diagnosis in which a definite anatomic or chemical test can be established. This trend, however, has led to alienation from the true clinical approach of direct unbiased observation, and still further away from effective therapy.

About forty years ago Poncet in Lyon established the theory that chronic arthritis must be caused by tubercle bacilli, a doctrine that was reanimated later on by Reitter and Loewenstein in Vienna. These authors claimed to have found tubercular bacilli in the blood of nearly every arthritic patient by a special method of culture. But this could not be confirmed by other investigators.

In the course of time *every new-fangled doctrine* such as endocrinology, allergy, vitamins, has been applied to explain the most varying diseases and among them also rheumatism and arthritism. But usually it has soon been found that the primary enthusiasm was too precipitate. This should make educated physicians more cautious and lead them back to the established traditional facts proved by practical success.

The present state of the problem of arthritis during the last thirty years

(In Europe and in America)

If we wish to get a quick survey of the changes in the problem of arthritis and allied conditions during the last thirty years and of the present state of this subject, it seems to us most practical to compare the leading textbooks of internal medicine in this era with the publications of recent years.

One of the most representative and widespread textbooks of internal medicine in Europe was that of Struempell (Leipzig and Vienna, 24th edition, 1922).

In reading Struempell's book we get the impression that there speaks a clinician of universal medical background such as is rarely found today. He speaks as a physician who is not over-specialized, and who does not give in to every new fashionable tendency and slogan.

However, as was characteristic of most clinicians of the last eighty years, (e.g., Cushing and Osler in America), Struempell, too, was influenced preponderantly by the anatomic trend. Significantly, he discussed in his textbook acute and chronic arthritis in the chapter on diseases of the organs of locomotion, whereas acute and chronic gout were treated among the metabolic diseases.

But as a matter of fact *chronic gout* and *chronic arthritis* very often *cannot be* distinguished or *separated,* as many transitions exist, still more complicated by various factors of etiology, individual constitution, and localization.

Struempell admitted that in spite of the enormous frequency of the disease our knowledge of the essence and the causes of chronic arthritis is still very meager. Very significantly he stated that the *infectious* cases are *rare* in proportion to the large majority of chronic cases. Furthermore, he believed that some general factors may induce acute as well as chronic arthritis, namely frequent colds, draft, drenching, living and working in damp, cold rooms in newly built houses, and certain professions such as laundress, etc. Therefore chronic arthritis also was called "arthritis of the poor" in contrast to acute gout, the arthritis of the glutton.

But Struempell overlooked that by far the most frequent form is the arthritis of the middle-aged, and in women arthritis of the menopause occurs in all ranks of society equally.

In contrast to the exaggerated up-to-date tendency to classify and separate many possibly exact subdivisions of arthritis, Struempell rightly stated that a clear-cut separation is impossible between the milder form of chronic arthritis, involving mostly the soft parts, and destructive arthritis (arthritis deformans) as an anatomic rather than etiologic conception.

As a practical-minded physician and as a constructive thinker, Struempell stressed more the common features of the different forms of arthritis, and also the common positive factors of therapy.

Concerning focal infection he said that such cases sometimes may occur, but not very frequently.

This coincides with our own experience that as a maximum not more than 5 to 10 per cent of all cases of chronic arthritis are infectious or even probably infectious in origin.

Very important is his statement that frequently chronic constitutional causes are present, primarily uric-acid diathesis and true gout. He also admitted that chronic arthritis and chronic gout may form *inseparable conditions,* and he also supposed endogenous causes such as endocrine factors. He considered chronic arthritis preponderantly a disease of mature and old age.

Other authors of this period distinguished between infectious "arthritis" and noninfectious "arthrosis."

The whole *gravity of our responsibility* and the imminent urgency of a more active and effective treatment of arthritis is revealed in the following much *too pessimistic* conclusions of Struempell, which correspond with those of almost all other modern clinicians. He said: "The *prognosis* of chronic polyarthritis and arthritis deformans, therefore, has to be called an *unfavorable* one. *Cures,* if they ever occur, can be performed very *rarely,* and only in the early stages."

A glance into the textbooks of earlier physicians and into my own records and those of my associates shows how *unjustified* this pessimistic outlook is.

Struempell continued: "However, it is favorable that the disease progresses so slowly, that the general condition, if we abstain from the local complaints, may be a bearable one for a very long time. Somewhat better is the prognosis in which only the soft parts of the joints are involved. However, here, too, cures are by no means frequent, and the gradual development of severe crippling changes in the joints is always to be feared."

I have quoted these sentences of one of the most experienced and leading clinicians of Europe so extensively, in order to demonstrate this modern *generally accepted pessimistic viewpoint,* clearly and completely.

Such a statement is important, because some authors still claim that physical therapy, vaccine, salicylates, sedatives, and treatment in the spas give sufficiently good results.

Concerning therapy Struempell recommended the compounds of salicylic acid, although he has "seen real advantage from it only seldom." More often he saw improvement by such alteratives as atophan, arsenic, iodine, iron, quinine, and codliver oil. Protein injections or chemotherapy may also bring about favorable response in some cases, but "one should not expect too much." Physical therapy, bathing, irritant or sedative liniments are also advised.

The most important and most effective form of local treatment, namely, draining of the skin by counter-irritation, is not mentioned at all, in accordance with the trend of the time.

Finally, arthritis of the spine was not subdivided by Struempell into different species, but the cure of this disease is considered impossible. In contrast with this widespread pessimistic view, my associates and I could and still can demonstrate many cases of arthritis of the spine in which the patients could drop their braces within a very short time and remain free of complaints.

A comprehensive monograph on this subject was written by E. Freund, head of the department of physical therapy at Wenckebach's Internal Clinic in Vienna, in 1929, under the title of *Joint Diseases*. According to the trend of the time, Freund believed that the main cause of chronic arthritis is infection, which, as we know now, was an error. On the other hand, Freund as well as other authors such as Trousseau, Charcot, and Pribram noted the striking *preference* of arthritis for the *female sex* at the rate of about four to one, (i.e., 80 per cent), and sometimes even six to one. This proportion increases in the higher brackets of age, so we may speak of arthritis of the *menopause* as an almost regular symptom. We may even speak of a sex-bound arthritis in women.

This is the reason why I, as a gynecologist and endocrinologist, as mentioned above, feel entitled to write on this subject, using also my experience in constitutional therapy of the female. According to Freund, the frequency of arthritis reaches its maximum in the fifth to the sixth decades of life.

Following his view, stressing infection, the *prognosis* of chronic arthritis usually is considered *unfavorable*. Some authors even speak of "progressive arthritis." The disease may stop by itself in every stage, but may leave behind deformation, stiffness, and restriction of mobility. Freund too, stressed the difficulty in separating chronic gout from chronic arthritis and from destructive arthritis. Characteristically his illustrations concerning arthritis deformans of the knee and hip joints displayed only female patients.

The treatment suggested is focal disinfection, physical therapy, bathing and protein or fever therapy. Hormonal treatment with ovarian substances have been disappointing.

Some authors have tried again to subdivide this condition. Thus the gynecologist Menge spoke of "arthropathia ovaripriva" after surgical or X-ray castration. Munk described an endocrine "arthritis sicca." Umber spoke of endogenous destructive periarthritis, concerning exclusively the female sex, and with no relation to any infection.

Heberden's nodes are considered a distinct disease but we have seen it so often combined with the usual form of polyarthritis in the menopause that it is rather arbitrary to see any essential difference, although Heberden's nodes are usually painless.

That the present trend toward the solving of problems mainly in exact analytic laboratory research often leads to *unnecessary pessimism,* we may also learn from the book of L. Lichtwitz, *Pathology of the Functions and Regulations* (New York, 1939).

The book is lavishly illustrated with curves, diagrams, figures, X-ray pictures, and laboratory findings. It attempts a synthesis between laboratory work and bedside, but it neglects completely the clinical experience of earlier physicians and effective therapy. Consequently Lichtwitz arrives at the end of his chapter on rheumatism at the following pessimistic conclusions:

"Vaccines, protein therapy, injections of sulfur have disappointed. The removal of foci by and large has achieved nothing, as many statistics of critical observers report in conformity. It is impossible to reconciliate the devil of rheumatism by hecatombs of tonsils and teeth. Dietetic treatment had no decisive influence.

"Physical therapy with individual dosage may be beneficial in correcting damages of the locomotive organs, and improving general health. Alteration from sensibility to immunity cannot yet be achieved. How this can be done, remains absolutely obscure."

The established and most effective practical therapy of *elimination* and *counter-irritation* as the most decisive factor has *not* been *mentioned* at all.

Effective unofficial cures of arthritis and allied conditions in the Nineteenth and Twentieth Centuries

What happened to all these very effective traditional methods of treating arthritis, rheumatism and allied conditions during the last hundred years? Did they disappear entirely? We have seen in the historical section how *many ways* earlier physicians of all times and nations had *to help* the sick, suffering from arthritis, sciatica, neuralgia, and rheumatism. With the abolition of traditional humoral pathology by Virchow, all these *established methods,* such as purging, bleeding, vomiting, sweating, and draining of the skin through counter-irritation were *discarded* as outmoded, useless, and even dangerous. Instead of these procedures, proved in practice, *nihilism* and resignation took their place, and arthritis with its allied conditions became a stepchild of medicine. Such patients were and still are often told that because we do not know the true cause of these conditions, there is no specific cure or *no cure* at all available.

This apparently logical but practically entirely wrong conclusion has been strikingly *refuted* by numerous medical *outsiders* and lay healers. Particularly in Europe there were many who attracted a large crowd of patients suffering from arthritis and rheumatism, who had been disappointed by official scientific or "school" medicine. These medical outsiders and quacks have successfully used different kinds of nostrums, mostly effective counter-irritants, and although they kept their remedies secret, their success in many cases that had been abandoned by the medical profession was and still is beyond any doubt.

It is easy to frown at these healers and call them quacks. I have preferred not to be hypocritical and to learn from them as much as I could. In doing so, I found myself in very good company. No less a man than Hippocrates stated that "one should not abhor asking the simple folks, [even the "quacks"] whether a thing is a good remedy, as many drugs have been found often enough by plain people and by mere chance rather than by planned scientific investigation."

Paracelsus, too, claimed on numerous occasions that he acquired many of his most effective remedies from lay healers of different walks of life such as barber surgeons, midwives, hangmen, gypsies, and herb-collecting old women. After all, as we have pointed out in the historical section, many of our most precious drugs had been used centuries previously by uneducated natives of different continents.

Ambroise Paré, who himself started not as a learned physician but as a barber surgeon, admitted that he tried to learn as much as possible from all available sources. Only recently Dr. H. E. Sigerist wrote on Paré's effective treatment of burns with fresh onions, which the latter had learned by chance from laymen.

Convinced of the frequent efficacy of these unofficial cures, I investigated them for many years and finally found that they are neither a secret nor a mere fraud, but nothing more or less than the *remnants of the classic tradition* thrown out the window by pedantic scientists and utilized by medical outsiders not only to their own benefit but also to that of otherwise helpless patients.

I have told the story of how in Vienna, in 1908, I became acquainted with Dr. Jetel's method of counter-irritation by which numerous cases of lumbago, sciatica, neuralgia, and arthritis were cured by artificial rash.

A similar method was used in Treviso near Venice, Italy, by Dr. Munari, who had his own large private clinic where thousands of otherwise discouraged patients from all over Europe were cured in a relatively short time. These patients were no superstitious fools, but mostly persons who had consulted the most outstanding medical authorities of Europe in vain.

A number of other counter-irritant, rash-producing liniments were used by different lay healers throughout Europe. Prominent among them was the Catholic priest Monsignor Kneipp, living in the small town of Woerishofen near Munich. As a reaction against the therapeutic nihilism on one hand and on the other hand, the surgical radicalism ruling during the second half of the nineteenth century, and partly even in our century, he preached simple diet, hydrotherapy, and the use of herbs improving the metabolism. He also used a strong counter-irritant containing croton oil, but he kept its detailed composition secret, for the treatment of arthritis and rheumatism. He scored numerous successes where official medicine failed. There were many lay healers of smaller caliber, particularly in Austria, Germany, and Switzerland, who made fortunes, and, although often persecuted by the medical authorities, still attracted a large crowd and often helped them.

We may refer to a case in which a woman was cured of a stiff knee joint by an artificial ulcer applied by such a country quack. In Vienna we had a simple postman who founded his own healing society, and his success, too, was based on such an effective counter-irritant.

Finally, we may remember a country quack near Graz in Styria (Austria) who cured arthritic patients with herbal decoctions, among them an important patient of mine who had consulted all available medical authorities of Vienna for her polyarthritis in vain. The country quack freed her of pain and restored her mobility within three weeks.

I could continue this list indefinitely. But all these experiences point to the fact that *we should study* and utilize the *writings* and experiences *of earlier physicians* as thoroughly as possible. The previous system of humoral pathology provides much more effective help to and also a better understanding of arthritis and allied conditions than does our preponderantly analytic, scholastic, and one-sided pedantic laboratory medicine. The exaggerated drive to be "exact and scientific" often narrows the horizon and leads to rigid dogmatism.

As I have pointed out in a recent article, "Empiricism and Rationalism in Past and Present Medicine" (*Bull. of the Hist. of Med.*, March, 1945), a permanent struggle always exists between these two trends. At present we are living in an era of extreme dogmatic and intolerant rationalism, banning the majority of all effective empirical methods that have been collected by our medical predecessors throughout the centuries, and thus impoverishing greatly our healing capacity. Present medicine is much too highbrow, hyperscientific, and more eager to provide "scientific evidence" and rationalistic explanations than to help the sick by all available means, even if the employed methods are "only empirical."

The United States is a great country, providing more freedom to its population than other nations. But we are sorry to say that in the field of modern medicine there is less freedom of thinking and more dogmatism than in any other field of human occupation.

With the best intentions of being progressive, realistic, and scientifically accurate, medical thought at present has become rigid, intolerant, narrow, mechanistic, bureaucratic, and reactionary. The medical student nowadays has to cram into his brain an enormous number of so-called exact but often unrelated and unnecessary facts and he does not dare to think or to speculate on higher guiding principles, because *medical systems, methodology,* and *philosophy* have been *expelled triumphantly* from medical education during the last hundred years. The result is mere technical routine and sticking to the "accepted" textbooks and views of medical schools, committees, and hospital staffs.

It was only recently that E. Moschowitz (Mount Sinai Hospital, New York) deplored the "too mechanistic" approach of our medical schools.

We had similar conditions in Europe where very often clinical assistants did not dare to air their own opinions if they were in contrast to the almighty head of the clinic who could influence their whole future.

Here in the United States, fortunately, there is in general less servility in the large clinics and hospitals, but the fear of being opposed to the "accepted" scientific views of medical authorities, medical schools, and committees is still much too widespread.

"Conformity" as a result of the votes of the majority is still overwhelming. This may be adequate in politics, but not in science.

It often looks as though nowadays one would make a fanatical religion out of science, which already borders on superstition. A new dogmatism, caused by misinterpretation and exaggerated application of the dead natural sciences (physics, chemistry, anatomy, etc.) to the living human organism rules at present. A more openminded study of medical *history* and *philosophy* would bring about more flexible thinking and a *more liberal approach* to many urgent problems, which seem to be caught in a deadlock. Arthritis and allied conditions as here treated provide just one, though one of the most drastic and striking examples, among many others.

ABOUT THE AUTHOR

BERNARD ASCHNER, M.D. is internationally recognized as a leading authority in the treatment of arthritis and rheumatism. He is a graduate of the University of Vienna and was on the staff of the Surgical University Clinic and at the Gynecological University Clinic in Vienna. In addition Dr. Aschner is recognized as a pioneer in the field of endocrinology. In 1908 he discovered the Oculocardiac Reflex (known in this country as Aschner's Phenomenon) and, in the same year, accomplished the first successful total removal of the pituitary gland in young dogs demonstrating (what was unknown before) that this gland is an indispensable organ for growth, sexual development and metabolism.

From 1918 to 1938 Dr. Aschner carried on an extensive clinical and private practice of international scope in surgery, obstetrics, women's diseases and arthritis. He is the originator and developer of a system of medicine known as Constitutional Therapy which has been accepted as a contribution of first theoretical and practical importance. He has lectured extensively before medical societies both in the U.S. and abroad.

Dr. Aschner has made his home in the U.S. since 1938. He was the Head of the Outpatient Department for Arthritis at Stuyvesant Polyclinic and at Lebanon Hospital in New York. He is a member of the New York Rheumatism Association, the American Medical Association, the Medical Society of the County of New York, and of the American Society for the History of Medicine. At present in addition to his private practice, he is continuing active research in the field of arthritis.

"THE MORE NATURAL OUR FOOD THE BETTER OUR HEALTH"

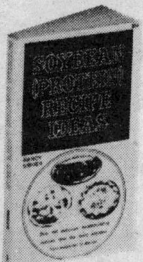 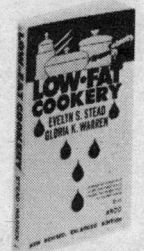 

SOYBEAN (PROTEIN) RECIPE IDEAS
Nancy Snider

As a major source of protein soybeans are a nutritious and endlessly versatile food. Here are over 100 unusual and delicious recipes that take the zesty soybean from breakfast to dinner in a fabulous cookbook by a noted home economist and food editor. Scores of diet and dollar stretching recipes—all easy to prepare and serve—and all featuring soy protein—soy stroganoff, meat loaf, soy breakfast items, soups, entrees, side dishes, sandwiches, breads, desserts, much more. Includes menu ideas and tips on cooking with soy.

Illustrated, **95¢**

LOW-FAT COOKERY
Evelyn S. Stead and Gloria K. Warren

Here finally is the perfect cookbook for a calorie-conscious, health-happy age. Incorporating more than 250 delicious, easy-to-follow recipes, **Low-Fat Cookery** puts the fun into dietetic cooking—and even more imporant, dietetic eating. Imagine delicious low-fat recipes for baked lasagna, fruitcake, bleu-cheese dressing, butterscotch sauce and lobster newburg. Included are invaluable aids to dietetic cooking with an easy-to-remember summary of the basic points of low-fat cookery, how to modify any recipe to obtain a low-fat content, information about new food products to enrich and diversify a low-fat diet, and a helpful discussion of special diets such as restricted sodium and unsaturated vegetable oil plans. **$1.65**

NATURE'S OWN VEGETABLE COOKBOOK
Ann Williams-Heller

Over 350 mouthwatering vegetable recipes—complete with practical information on the buying, storing, cooking, seasoning and nutritional value of each vegetable. With this cookbook, noted nutritionist Ann Williams-Heller has opened the door to an entirely new culinary world. She brings her cooking genius to bear on every available vegetable—in main dishes, casseroles, salads, soups and their countless variations. Also included are recipes for sauces and salad dressings as well as nutrition charts that show the vitamin and mineral content of each vegetable. **$1.45**

BLUEPRINTS FOR BETTER HEALTH

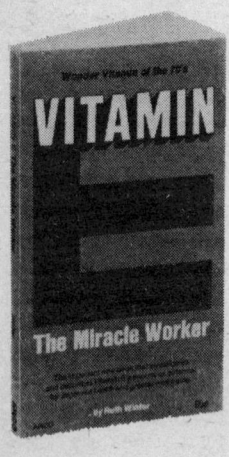

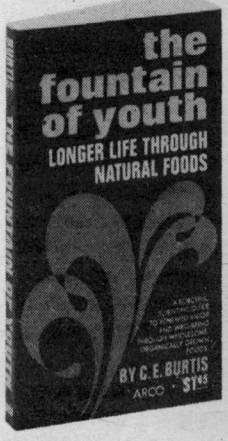

VITAMIN E—
THE MIRACLE WORKER

Ruth Winter

A simple, scientifically sound and comprehensive book that presents all the facts regarding the superb properties and marvelous potential of Vitamin E. Ruth Winter, a respected medical writer, examines the many claims and counter claims made for this extraordinary vitamin and reveals its reported usefullness in fighting infertility, ulcers and arthritis, its importance in preventing blood clots, its effectiveness against heart disease, cancer in animals and its significant role in retarding the aging process. Essential reading for everyone concerned about their own health and the health of their loved ones. **95¢**

THE FOUNTAIN OF YOUTH

C.E. Burtis

A thorough guide to renewed vigo and well-being through wholesom organically grown foods, combine with a startling, fully documente expose of the adulterants and de structive processing that poiso much of our daily fare. Based o a lifetime of research and exper mentation in the field of nutritio Mr. Burtis' book shows exact how wholesome natural foods ca bring renewed youth, vitality, fi ness and the priceless gift of longer life. Here are menus easy-to-prepare health foods a eating methods that assure t best digestion and fullest use a food's nourishing qualities well as a discussion of dangero foods. **$1.**

THESE TWO BOOKS
COULD CHANGE YOUR LIFE

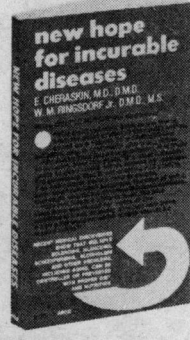 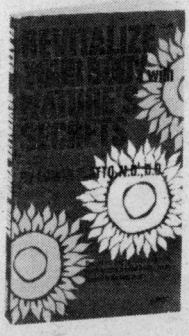

NEW HOPE FOR INCURABLE DISEASES

E. Cheraskin, M.D. and
W.M. Ringsdorf, Jr., M.D.

The revolutionary bestseller that proves in simple, everyday language that the battle against many dread diseases previously considered hopeless is being won—today. Stressing simple organic improvements in diet and nutrition and recent dramatic discoveries in these areas, the authors outline radically new and hopeful treatments for some of the most feared ailments of our time—multiple sclerosis, glaucoma, heart disease, mental retardation, birth defects and others. "It is likely to become the most valuable guide to good health anyone could posess . . . an historic book, a must for all health seekers. The material on food supplements alone, is worth the price of the book." — Better Nutrition $1.65

REVITALIZE YOUR BODY WITH NATURE'S SECRETS

Edwin Flatto, N.D., D.O.

A respected homeopathic physician explores every aspect of physical and mental well-being, never losing sight of the fact that health is the natural state of the body while disease is an unnatural state of imbalance. Fasting as a way to cleanse the body of toxic waste, the importance of a diet of wholesome, natural foods and the rewards of right eating are covered, as are exercise as therapy and the health benefits of fresh air and sunshine. Scores of questions on the problems of overweight, ulcers, varicose veins, acne, sinus trouble, constipation, colds and other common ailments are answered. Soundly scientific, easy-to-follow, this simple book promises lasting health, undreamed vigor and the happiness and peace that go with them.

$1.45

"THE MORE NATURAL OUR FOOD THE BETTER OUR HEALTH"

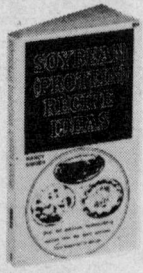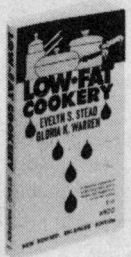

SOYBEAN (PROTEIN) RECIPE IDEAS
Nancy Snider

As a major source of protein soybeans are a nutritious and endlessly versatile food. Here are over 100 unusual and delicious recipes that take the zesty soybean from breakfast to dinner in a fabulous cookbook by a noted home economist and food editor. Scores of diet and dollar stretching recipes—all easy to prepare and serve—and all featuring soy protein—soy stroganoff, meat loaf, soy breakfast items, soups, entrees, side dishes, sandwiches, breads, desserts, much more. Includes menu ideas and tips on cooking with soy.

Illustrated, **95¢**

LOW-FAT COOKERY
Evelyn S. Stead and Gloria K. Warren

Here finally is the perfect cookbook for a calorie-conscious, health-happy age. Incorporating more than 250 delicious, easy-to-follow recipes, **Low-Fat Cookery** puts the fun into dietetic cooking—and even more imporant, dietetic eating. Imagine delicious low-fat recipes for baked lasagna, fruitcake, bleu-cheese dressing, butterscotch sauce and lobster newburg. Included are invaluable aids to dietetic cooking with an easy-to-remember summary of the basic points of low-fat cookery, how to modify any recipe to obtain a low-fat content, information about new food products to enrich and diversify a low-fat diet, and a helpful discussion of special diets such as restricted sodium and unsaturated vegetable oil plans. **$1.45**

NATURE'S OWN VEGETABLE COOKBOOK
Ann Williams-Heller

Over 350 mouthwatering vegetable recipes--complete with practical information on the buying, storing, cooking, seasoning and nutritional value of each vegetable. With this cookbook, noted nutritionist Ann Williams-Heller has opened the door to an entirely new culinary world. She brings her cooking genius to bear on every available vegetable—in main dishes, casseroles, salads, soups and their countless variations. Also included are recipes for sauces and salad dressings as well as nutrition charts that show the vitamin and mineral content of each vegetable. **$1.45**

HEALTH and MEDICINE BOOKS